This book is dedicated to more than 50 percent of the

U.S. population, those who are struggling with their weight

and the medical complications resulting from it.

We hope this book will offer a first step.

CONTENTS

Contents

Introduction

"YOU'RE FAT BECAUSE you eat too much. Why don't you just eat less?"

"Your lipids are high because you don't exercise enough and you eat too much fat. Why don't you control your eating and get off your duff?"

"If you didn't eat so much junk food, you wouldn't have all those problems. Why don't you stop going to all those drive-throughs?"

How often have you heard those words?

Or stories like these:

"I was downright skinny as a child, normal or chubby as an adolescent, and trim as an adult. But I have a family history of obesity. They weren't always fat. It seemed that at about age forty, the weight started to appear, and then, by their mid- to late fifties, most of the people on my mother's side had developed type 2 diabetes or heart trouble and all the medical complications that follow. Generally their last few years were no bed of roses.

"At age forty, I was eight pounds heavier than my trim adult weight at age twenty. I was also a smoker. At age forty-two, weighing 172 pounds, I gave up smoking—cold turkey. That was December 2, 1986. By the following Christmas, I weighed 192 pounds with a cholesterol level of 240 mg/dL and a miserable HDL of 29 mg/dL."

That is the biographical information of one of the creators of this diet. For the other, it was a history of weight gain beginning after age forty, despite adherence to the USDA Food Pyramid and low-fat foods and exercise.

"I ran until I got a stress fracture of my tibia, but the weight crept up each year."

We both exercised. We both ate appropriately according to the standards of various health organizations. We both followed exactly what we had been taught, and yet, we were getting fatter every year. Was our heredity to blame? Were we, like so many Americans, simply fated by our genes?

Even worse—we both work in health care. We were giving other people the same advice that had failed for us. It didn't seem right.

In 1996, we decided there was only one way to approach the epidemic of weight gain in which we were entrapped: scientifically. We collaborated on an in-depth review of the available scientific literature concerning weight loss and improvement in serum lipids through the use of diet. We also looked at the popular diets being touted at the time.

Although no one diet was ideal, there were facets of many that were actually good ideas, with science to support them. Looking further into the subspecialty literature allowed us to find clinical trials that tested single dietary components in patients who had diseases that were made worse by obesity. Slowly, we extracted evidence that low-carbohydrate diets could result in weight loss.

But what about the rest of the dietary components: fats and their composition, proteins, and macro- and micronutrients? The diabetes literature demonstrated that diets high in monounsaturated fats and fiber could improve glycemic control. The preventative medicine and oncology and infectious disease literature added information about natural sources of vitamins, almost miraculous phytochemicals and micronutrients, probiotics, and dietary fiber.

Things were coming together. Perhaps a safe diet could be designed that would enhance weight loss and weight maintenance and at the same time promote good health. Besides, weight was not the sole issue faced by Americans. There are other diseases—prostate and breast cancer, asthma, coronary artery disease, hypertension, stroke, type 2 diabetes—that may be affected by poor dietary choices, and the incidences of some of these diseases are rising. Wouldn't promoting health and preventing disease with one comprehensive plan serve us best?

We developed what we called the Goldberg-O'Mara Diet—the GO-Diet for short—in 1996 and promptly put ourselves on it as the first subjects, studying its effects on our blood chemistries and weight. Dr. Goldberg lost twelve pounds in the first month. Dr. O'Mara began just before Halloween and was twenty-five pounds lighter that Christmas.

Introduction

Laboratory studies confirmed its safety. By May 1997, we started our formal studies in moderately to severely obese volunteers and later reported its success. Subsequently, hundreds of people, informally or with their doctors, have used the diet published in our first book, *GO-Diet: The Goldberg-O'Mara Diet Plan*.

In the ensuing years, our diet has evolved further, emphasizing the wealth of scientific literature that has been published on diet composition and its impact on health. The basic elements are the same as in 1996, and the four cornerstones that make the diet safe and effective are stronger than ever. But because the diet's four main elements are critical to its success, we decided to choose a new name for the diet—one that emphasizes the four components and their impact on overall health. Hence the new name: the Four Corners Diet.

For this diet to be safe and effective, you must choose foods daily from each of the "four corners": low net carbohydrates, high fiber, high monounsaturated fats, and what we call pharmafoods.

Pharmafoods is a term we're using for foods that are so healthy, they have an almost pharmaceutical effect when included in your diet. Their natural composition includes substances that have health-promoting—and, possibly, disease-preventing—effects. They're just too good for you not to include them in your diet every day.

We encourage you to try the diet for just three months. If you're like our original study's moderately to severely obese subjects, you will see an average loss of twenty pounds of weight and five inches off your waist, as well as improved total cholesterol and triglyceride levels. If your weight is normal, you will see metabolic improvements and perhaps sense an increase in energy.

This diet is not just for weight loss. It can also help people with diabetes, especially those with type 2 diabetes, who tend to be overweight. Type 2 diabetes has reached epidemic proportions in the United States. It is linked to obesity in both adults and children. The Four Corners Diet may be of particular use for those who have this disease. If you have type 2 diabetes, you should see a dramatic improvement in your blood-glucose control and lipid levels as well as a loss of weight.

In this edition of our book, we have invited Gretchen Becker—the author of *The First Year—Type 2 Diabetes* and *Stop Diabetes: 50 Simple Steps You Can Take at Any Age to Reduce Your Risk of Type 2 Diabetes*—to add insights on the use of this diet by people with type 2 diabetes. She has written the *If You Have Diabetes* sections of the book, as well as

Chapter 11. Although these sections are designed primarily for people with type 2 diabetes, who are usually overweight, a healthy low-carbohydrate diet may also benefit those with type 1 diabetes, because lower carbohydrate intake results in smaller blood sugar swings and less need for insulin.

Becker also performed the nutritional analyses with the aid of the Computer Planned Menus program from Nutritional Computing Concepts and followed the suggested menus for a week to make sure they were reasonable. She was not involved in developing the diet, however, and when we use the term *we* in this book, we mean the two originators of the diet, Drs. Goldberg and O'Mara.

Becker has personal experience with diabetes. She was diagnosed with the disease in 1996 and was told to follow the low-fat, calorie-restricted American Diabetes Association diet. She did lose weight on this diet, but she was hungry twenty-four hours a day, constantly thinking about her next meal, and decided this was not a way she could live for the rest of her life. In addition, her blood sugar levels were too high.

Hence she slowly started eating fewer carbohydrates and more healthy fats in nuts and olive oil and ended up with a diet very similar to the Four Corners Diet. Her blood sugar levels improved, her constant hunger disappeared, the weight she had lost stayed off (she is now in the normal range for body mass index), and she decided this was a healthy diet for a lifetime, especially for people with type 2 diabetes.

"There are other low-carbohydrate diets out there that help people with type 2 diabetes get their blood sugar levels under control," she said. "But many low-carb diets are high in saturated fat and low in calcium and fiber. I don't know of any other low-carb diet that has such an emphasis on healthy foods and healthy fats, as well as fiber and cultured milk products."

All three authors find the Four Corners Diet a satisfying way of eating that they plan to follow for the rest of their lives. Why don't you give it a try and see if it will work for you, too?

TABLE 1.1
The Four Corners Diet in a Nutshell

LOW CARBOHYDRATES Up to 50 grams of net carbohydrate per day Up to 15 grams of net carbohydrate per meal	**HIGH MONOUNSATURATED FAT** 50 percent of fat as heart-healthy monounsaturated
HIGH FIBER 25 to 30 grams of fiber per day	**PHARMAFOODS** Probiotics every day Other pharmafoods every day

Because changes in your diet can dramatically alter your metabolism, you should consult your doctor if you take any prescription medication whenever you change your diet in any way. We recommend seeing your doctor for a weigh-in, blood pressure check, and basic lipid and metabolic screen before you begin the diet, and then again after eight to twelve weeks to gauge its effect on you.

THE
FOUR CORNERS
DIET

ONE

It Worked for Them

"**N**ONE OF THE other diets I had attempted changed me like this one did," said Berry L., MD, who describes himself as a "big guy," an ex-athlete who ballooned up to 325 pounds after major surgery forced him to be inactive in a leg cast for six weeks.

"By avoiding rice, pasta, and bread, I found myself eating all of the foods that I desire and was surprised to find that the pounds began to come off and stay off," despite the fact that he had just quit smoking.

Dr. L. also noticed a change in his appetite on the Four Corners Diet. "One amazing discovery while I was in the early phases of this diet was that I was never hungry. Though restricting my carbohydrate intake, I was still able to eat enough food to be full and satisfied. One of the benefits of lowering one's insulin level is that you find that you don't have the fluctuations in your appetite or cravings. And consequently, I now eat even smaller portions than before."

Dr. L. is not alone. We have seen many people in the Chicago area benefit from the Four Corners Diet. In our formal study of the diet, described in detail in Chapter 12, the average weight loss was twenty pounds in twelve weeks.

Because the volunteers were mainly employees at the hospital in which we both worked, we were able to follow their success as their weight loss continued after the study period. The original group recruited even more of their friends and families, and of course we gave the diet freely to anyone who asked. So we heard a lot of success stories and actually watched the process in many others.

It was so nice to see the technician who was 200 pounds get down to 135 pounds over nine months. It was good to hear about the diabetic sister of one of our study participants who went on the diet with her doctor's supervision. She went from using 95 units of insulin daily to using an oral agent only. We were thrilled when one woman lost 25 pounds—the first time in her life that she had been able to lose any weight at all.

Then there was one of our doctors, who threw out five progressively smaller belts in six months as he shed 56 pounds. He now proudly wears his shirts tucked in, whereas he used to wear only loose scrub tops to work.

Since then, we have been pleased to see that many of these hospital employees have managed to *keep the weight off* since the diet's inception in 1996. This is because the Four Corners Diet is, as Karen C. said, "more than a diet. It is a healthy, sensible way of eating." Karen was unable to lose the 12 pounds she had gained with the birth of her last child until she tried the Four Corners Diet, and "I dropped the weight immediately and have kept it off effortlessly for six months," she said. "My husband has lost 32 pounds and counting."

"This is not a diet, it's a way of life, or just healthy eating," said Phil G., who dropped his triglycerides from 700 to 150 by following the diet.

Others have referred to the long-term lifestyle change that occurred with the Four Corners Diet. "This diet really changed my life," said Dr. L. "The 'craving' for all those extra carbohydrates actually does go away, and as a big guy it is a pleasure to eat primarily meats and fresh vegetables and fresh salads daily. Instead of starting the day with loads of coffee and doughnuts, I eat a balanced breakfast of omelets and a half cup of fruit."

But this diet results in more than weight loss. It improves your health and sense of well-being as well. There is also no question about its effects on people's sense of energy. Many people said it had become a habit to sneak a nap at around four or five o'clock in the afternoon. They attributed this phenomenon to their age or workload or stress levels. Yet, almost without exception, the need for an afternoon nap completely disappeared within a week of starting the diet. People said that the diet gave them ten years back. And this decreased need for naps predated any serious loss of weight or inches.

"Not only did the pounds slip away with ease, but I suddenly felt and even looked more alive," said Kathy G. "I suddenly had more energy, and I began needing less sleep each night. I also no longer felt like falling asleep after my midday and evening meals anymore. This diet is a lifestyle change—for the better."

We now laugh about it, yet we were previously resigned to "needing" extra rest. Changing our diet away from excessive carbohydrates had an impact upon our "need" for extra daytime sleep, and with it went the concept that we were just getting older and needed naps.

Of course, the psychological benefits of weight loss are unbeatable for self-esteem. We see turtlenecks being worn under lab coats now, something it was impossible to do when there was a fat layer protruding. We and our fellow dieters have thrown out or given away dowdy clothes in favor of more trendy cuts and shorter hemlines. No one fears summer.

"Needless to say, my wife enjoys the fact that I look great," said Dr. L. "I'm sure she looks forward to a shared lifetime of the kind of physical and emotional stability this sustained weight loss has allowed."

In August 1998, our research was presented at a national meeting in Chicago. The local news station, Channel 2, picked up the story as part of their own series on diets. We were interviewed by Dr. Michael Breen, a highly respected physician-journalist who caught on to the concepts of the diet immediately. A very short segment of video was run on the news over the next couple of days. The response to the story was overwhelming. More than seventeen thousand people requested the diet after seeing the brief story on television. Copies of our diet were distributed, and we set up a Web site in order to reach more people. As part of our Web site, we set up a "virtual" support group. Between the Web site and mailings, we have received hundreds of testimonials from people who have started the diet.

Many of the stories followed the same theme. People had "dieted" for years, gradually becoming resigned to being overweight for life. Imagine their surprise when, for the first time, a diet actually produced weight loss without any penalties. People wrote to us about losing weight and buying new clothes for the first time in years, and in much lower dress sizes than they had ever expected! They told us of lowered weights and lowered cholesterol levels.

"It has lowered my cholesterol to normal (over one hundred points)," said Mary Fran M., "and truly, I don't crave the carbs."

They told us about having energy to do things after work. They told us about their new body images and feelings they now have about themselves.

"The best part about the diet (way of life) is that it is easy to understand, and when used with exercise, it maximizes your results," said Phil G., a young business professional who is still active in sports. "Now here is the great advantage. When not working out and still on the diet, it helps keep the muscle longer and protect what you've worked on in the past. This was a bonus for those busy times at work when I could not make it to the gym. The biggest surprise was the ability to have high energy and good physical appearance without the exercise when focused on the diet compared to only a great exercise schedule and no diet."

One of our casual dieters, an emergency physician at a busy Chicago-area hospital, started the diet in January 1998 and lost eighty pounds by the end of the year. During this time he also quit smoking (something he had done once before in the past) and was thrilled to find that he still lost weight instead of gaining it. His enthusiasm was catching. Several others in the emergency department started the diet as a result of seeing his success with it.

At the end of 1998, that emergency department had lost some serious weight. When we were asked to appear in February 1999 on WGN, Channel 9 in Chicago, they asked for someone who had been on the diet to share his story; the doctor was up for the challenge. The news team was skeptical of a high–monounsaturated fat, low-carbohydrate diet. Wasn't it going to be hard to follow? Wouldn't it use alien foods? Imagine their surprise when he made lunch for them: homemade Caesar salad and chicken cacciatore! The visit that was supposed to be just a few minutes lasted two and a half hours.

The news team learned that eating normal portions of the real foods—healthy foods—on the Four Corners Diet can result in serious weight loss. Hundreds of people have found that it worked for them. You can join them.

TWO

You Haven't Failed— Your Diets Have

I F YOU'RE OVERWEIGHT, you've undoubtedly been on diets before. Lots of them. Most of them worked, and you were able to lose some weight, maybe even significant amounts.

Then you got tired of feeling deprived all the time and started eating again just like everyone else. And all that weight came back, most likely even more than you'd lost. You were a victim of the famous yo-yo dieting cycle. Lose a little. Gain back even more. Lose a little more. Gain back even more. Lose a little more. You get the picture. Now you're heavier than you ever were before you started dieting.

Maybe you think you're a hopeless failure, you have a moral weakness, there's something wrong with your willpower, and you'll never be able to lose weight and keep it off. But consider this. Maybe there's nothing wrong with you. Instead, there's something wrong with the diets you've been following. They're simply not viable for long-term weight control.

Before we describe the Four Corners Diet, let's briefly review various weight-control practices that have been tried through the years.

Basically, two different nonsurgical approaches have been used: increased exercise and reduced calorie consumption.

Exercise is healthy, and it can help you keep from gaining more weight. But in order to lose weight through exercise alone, you'd have to do an awful lot of strenuous exercise. A pound of fat contains 3,500 calories, and a "brisk" walk burns only about 200 calories, more or less, depending on your size. So you'd have to go on almost eighteen such walks to lose even a pound, and that assumes that all that exercise didn't just make you hungrier. Most people won't lose more than four to seven pounds through exercise alone.

If you're severely obese, or if you have coronary artery disease or atherosclerosis or arthritis or other limiting medical conditions, the kind of exercise that would make you lose weight is simply not appropriate, or even possible.

The other approach is severe calorie restriction. Yes, almost everyone will lose weight when they take in very few calories. You don't see a lot of fat people in forced-labor camps or areas suffering from famine. But severe calorie restriction, meaning eating less than about 800 calories (depending on your size), can have serious consequences, including death. Less severe diets of 1,000 to 1,500 calories, often attained by eating only a few types of food—for example, grapefruit diets, cabbage diets, or rice diets, or sometimes only expensive liquid or other packaged foods—usually produce weight loss.

But how many people want to eat nothing but canned drinks or expensive trademarked diet TV dinners for the rest of their lives? Not many. When they reach their goal—often even before that point—they revert to their old eating habits and the weight returns.

Studies show that as much as two thirds of the weight lost through calorie-restrictive diets is often regained within a year. Almost all regain the weight by the end of five years. Even when behavioral modification techniques are used, most people will regain all the weight they lost within five years. Furthermore, weight loss through calorie restriction can result in the loss of muscle tissue in addition to—or in excess of—the loss of fat. Another problem with calorie-restricted diets is that you have difficulty getting sufficient vitamins and minerals when eating very small quantities of food, so nutritional supplements are needed.

Drastic approaches to reducing the number of calories you eat involve various surgical procedures. These include wiring the jaw to reduce the intake of solid foods; stapling the stomach to reduce its capacity; and inflating balloons in the stomach to create a sense of fullness.

Other techniques involve bypassing a portion of the intestine that absorbs a lot of nutrients so that many of them pass right through the body, in addition to reducing the size of the stomach. Such surgery also seems to affect the secretion of appetite-controlling hormones, so people who have had this surgery say they don't feel hungry—despite eating tiny meals.

Bypass surgery can result in significant weight loss—and also normalize blood sugar levels in people with type 2 diabetes. However, the resulting unnatural connection between stomach and intestine also interferes with the absorption of some essential nutrients such as vitamins, and people who have had this surgery must take supplements for the rest of their lives. Furthermore, any surgery carries risks of infection and death. In some people, the smaller stomach simply expands with time, and because they haven't learned new eating habits, the weight returns.

Some diets reduce calories by reducing specific food groups. One popular approach, endorsed by the U.S. Department of Agriculture through their Food Pyramid, as well as by groups such as the American Heart Association, the American Dietetic Association, and the American Diabetes Association, has been to restrict fat.

This is for two reasons. First, fat has more calories per gram than carbohydrate and protein, so the idea was that you could eat more food and get fewer calories. Second, many Americans have problems with abnormal levels of lipids (cholesterol and triglycerides) in their blood, and increased blood lipid levels are associated with heart disease.

Triglyceride is just a fancy name for *fat*. So the assumption was that if you ate less fat, the triglyceride levels in your blood would go down. There is also evidence that *saturated* fat in the diet makes your cholesterol levels go up.

So Americans started eating less fat. Food manufacturers jumped on the bandwagon and started offering reduced-fat and fat-free versions of most popular foods. And what happened? Americans got fatter than ever.

What went wrong? Well, first you have to understand that there are basically only three types of food: fat, protein, and carbohydrate. If you eat less fat, you have to eat more protein or carbohydrate. Most protein foods (meat and cheese, for example) also contain fat. So you can't eat a lot of meat on a low-fat diet. That means you've got to increase your consumption of carbohydrate—on some very low-fat diets up to 70 percent of your total day's food.

Second, carbohydrates are cheap. Food manufacturers were naturally thrilled with the idea that they could offer tempting snack foods that contained very little expensive protein and a lot of cheap starch. By making them salty and sugary and crispy and even addictive, they could sell a lot and reap huge profits. Some low-fat diet people said you could eat all the carbohydrates you wanted as long as you limited the fat, so people thought they could have as much of these fat-free foods as they wanted and ate even more calories in nonnutritious carby snack foods than they'd ever eaten before.

An additional problem with such diets is that triglycerides often *increase* on low-fat diets, especially those with a lot of processed carbohydrate foods.

Another approach to weight loss is exactly the opposite of the low-fat approach. This limits calories by limiting the amount of carbohydrates you eat. Various versions of such diets have been around for a long time, but in the recent past the most vocal champion of the low-carb diets was the late cardiologist Robert Atkins. He took a lot of flak from establishment groups such as the American Heart Association for his version of a low-carb diet, which called for liberal amounts of fat. The dieter was allowed to choose saturated fats if desired. Endocrinologist Richard Bernstein continues to be a champion of low-carb diets for people with diabetes.

These diets do work for most people, for reasons we'll explain later. And, counterintuitively, eating more fat, regardless of its type, seems to lower the levels of blood fats in most people when they also limit their intake of carbohydrates. However, about 30 percent of people who go on a high-saturated-fat version of a low-carb diet (more than 40 grams, or 1.4 ounces of saturated fat a day) do see their lipid levels get worse and hence may actually increase their cardiac risk factors at the same time they're losing weight. Also, although Atkins urged people to eat low-carb vegetables, they weren't required. Instead he prescribed complex, often expensive vitamin formulas for those following his plan.

It sounds as if no diet is perfect. Does that mean you should consider drugs instead? A variety of pharmacological approaches have been tried that either attempt to reduce your appetite or increase your metabolism, making you burn more of the calories you eat.

Diuretics (sometimes called water pills) make you lose water weight. But you can lose too much water, become dehydrated, and disrupt the balance of electrolytes in your blood. Unless you have congestive heart failure, you don't want to lose water; you want to lose fat.

Others have tried amphetamines, thyroid hormones, and other drugs that stimulate the sympathetic nervous system and increase your metabolic rate. They can also cause sleep deprivation and cardiac arrhythmias and can become addictive. Drugs that combine appetite suppressants with substances that stimulate the metabolic rate have been associated with a fatal form of heart disease called primary pulmonary hypertension. You may recall reading about a drug combination known as Fen-Phen (a combination of fenfluramine and phentermine) that originally seemed to be effective but turned out to be associated with these serious complications and was withdrawn from the market. Sibutramine (Meridia) is a drug that affects mood and also seems to reduce appetite. However, the increase in weight loss is only about ten pounds a year, and the drug has side effects such as constipation, insomnia, agitation, and increased blood pressure. Orlistat (Xenical) interferes with the absorption of fat, which is then excreted in the feces. Sounds great, but it also causes increased defecation and occasional oily "accidents" that are difficult to control. It also interferes with the absorption of fat-soluble vitamins. Someday the perfect weight-loss drug may be produced, and whoever makes it will undoubtedly become rich. But that time isn't now. The risk/benefit odds of today's drugs are simply not good.

How about psychological approaches to weight loss? Some people think all people with weight problems have a psychological need to eat. Maybe they're unhappy, lonely, or have low self-esteem. Or maybe they're obsessive, and the obsession focuses on food.

There are undoubtedly some people who do eat too much to satisfy deep psychological needs. For such people counseling may help. But as the news media seems to tell us every day, more than half of all Americans are overweight, and that many people are unlikely to have serious psychological disturbances. The American diet has simply become unhealthy. Almost all of us eat too much food and the wrong types of food.

We all lead busy lives that, unfortunately, mostly involve sedentary occupations; most of us don't do heavy, hard labor. We've become a service economy, not an agricultural or physical labor one. We drive to work or take public transportation; we don't walk. But most of all, we're busy. We think we don't have time to grow our own vegetables or even cut and chop fresh foods to make our own meals. We love convenience foods. We love to get soft drinks out of machines. We love to eat our meals at restaurants. And all of these convenience foods tend to be heavy on starches, including a lot of sugar, and saturated fat. Even fruits, which most people think of as health foods, have been engineered to be bigger, juicier, and sweeter than their earlier, now-heirloom counterparts. And remember that fruits used to be available only during short summer seasons. We can now eat them year-round. Fruit juices contain even more sugar, without the healthy fiber that slows down the digestion of the whole fruit.

For reasons we explain later, sugar consumption is one of the major contributors to weight gain. And when we say "sugar" we mean sugar in all its forms: table sugar (called sucrose), corn syrup (usually called high-fructose corn syrup in food labels), fruit sugar (fructose), milk sugar (lactose), grape sugar (glucose), and starch. "But starch isn't a sugar," you may think. You're right. But starch consists of chains of a sugar (glucose) linked together like a string of beads, and as soon as you eat it, your body breaks the starch down into sugar. So for all practical purposes, eating starch is the same as eating sugar. You can test this yourself by putting a bit of a cracker into your mouth and chewing for a while. Enzymes in your mouth break down the starch, and you should be able to taste the sweetness.

Limiting sugar in all its forms can help you to lose weight. It should also reduce your triglyceride levels and thus contribute to your cardiac health. Hence this is Corner 1 of the Four Corners Diet. But this diet doesn't stop there. There's more to healthy eating than limiting carbohydrates.

We also emphasize monounsaturated fats, which do not raise cholesterol levels. This is Corner 2.

Corner 3 is fiber, including natural unprocessed foods high in fiber, which is often lacking in other low-carb diets and whose benefits we will extol in later chapters.

Finally, Corner 4 is what we call pharmafoods, foods that have been shown to have health benefits beyond simply containing vitamins and minerals. These include the probiotic foods like yogurt and kefir, and other pharmafoods such as vegetables that are high in antioxidants and cancer-preventive phytochemicals (just a fancy word for plant chemicals).

Eating foods from each of the corners every day should not only help you lose weight—and if you have diabetes, control your blood sugar levels as well—but it should ensure that you get a healthy dose of vitamins, minerals, fiber, antioxidants, and other disease-preventive compounds every day without taking huge doses of artificial vitamins.

On the Four Corners Diet, you'll eat normal amounts of protein and normal amounts of calories. We repeat: *normal amounts of calories.* There is no need to count calories on this diet. We focus only on a few measurements—mostly carbohydrate, monounsaturated fat, and fiber.

Because you're not limiting your calories, the Four Corners Diet contains enough real food that you won't feel hungry. And it's varied enough that you shouldn't feel deprived and should be able to make it a way of eating for a lifetime—which is what you need if you're going to not only lose weight but *keep it off.*

Interested? If you're ready to get started, you can skip to Chapter 4. If you want to know a little more about why the Four Corners Diet works, the next chapter describes it in more detail.

▶ IF YOU HAVE DIABETES

EXERCISE ALONE MAY not contribute much to your weight loss, but it will do a great deal to help you control your blood sugar levels, so you should try to do as much as you are able.

We're not talking about running ten miles a day carrying fifty-pound weights here. Anything helps. If you're very overweight, just walking a block or two at first may be all that you're able to do. If you have arthritis or some other disabling condition, maybe chair exercises or gentle swimming is all that you can reasonably do. That's okay. Something is always better than nothing.

Exercise makes your muscles take up glucose (blood sugar) from the bloodstream without the aid of insulin. It also makes whatever insulin you're able to make yourself (or you inject) more effective. Thus exercise is a wonderful way to help keep your blood sugar levels down. In fact, if you're using insulin or one of the sulfonylurea drugs that make your body produce insulin, exercise could make your blood sugar levels go *too* low. So if you are using insulin or a sulfonylurea, speak with your doctor or diabetes educator to learn how to tell when you should and when you shouldn't exercise.

Exercise also increases the amount of muscle in your body, and muscle takes more glucose out of the blood than other tissues. Thus, the more muscle you have, the easier it should be for you to keep your blood sugar levels down. Exercise has a double benefit if you have diabetes.

THREE

Why Four Corners?

THE MAJORITY OF people who lose weight through dieting just regain it within a few years. Why? There may be several reasons. Some people think everyone has a set point, a weight at which your body wants to be, and that if dieting brings you below your set point, your metabolism will go down so much and your hunger will increase so much that you'll just regain everything you've lost. According to this theory, thin people have a low set point and fat people have a high set point. According to this theory, it's all hopeless. According to this theory, your genes are your destiny.

Genes undoubtedly do contribute to your weight. Some people have genes that let them eat all they want. You know the type. They sit opposite you at the cafeteria shoveling in carbohydrate-rich foods as well as fats, yet they are skinny. Not slim, but really skinny. It seems unfair, doesn't it. The rest of us will always have to be more careful with our diets. But we don't think the situation is hopeless. There are other reasons why most dieters eventually regain most of the weight they lose on diets.

One major reason is the word *diet*. Many people think of a diet as a temporary way of eating that will last only until they reach their goal weight. At that point they stop the diet and start eating "normally" again, according to their own definition of "normal." Unfortunately, it was eating normally that put the weight on in the first place. So naturally the weight returns.

This situation is almost certain to occur on any kind of artificial diet, such as severe calorie restriction, so dangerous that it can only be undertaken in a medical setting; even moderate calorie restriction with which you constantly feel deprived; a diet that involves meals in cans or bars or prepared expensive frozen dinners purchased from a diet company; or a diet, like the rice diet, that restricts you to only one or several types of foods, a situation that no one can tolerate for long.

For you to not only lose weight but keep it off, *your diet must be varied and nutritious enough that you can stick to it for the rest of your life.* You have to think of it not as a temporary diet that you'll stop when you reach your goal, but as a total restructuring of your approach to food, a way of eating that you'll *enjoy* without thinking of it as a diet.

The Four Corners diet does just that. If you follow this plan, you should lose your excess weight and then slow down the weight loss as you get close to your body's ideal weight. At that point, you don't change your way of eating and stop the diet. You just stick with it, and the weight should stay off. As Phil G. said in Chapter 1, "This is not a diet, it's a way of life."

The Four Corners diet is a low-carbohydrate diet. But eating low carb doesn't mean you'll have nothing but steak and cheese and eggs for the rest of your life. Remember, there are four corners to this diet, and low carb is only one. All four corners are important for your health. There are plenty of nutritious low-carb vegetables; probiotic foods like yogurt; nuts; low-carb breads and desserts; and high-fiber fruits that will fit into a low-carb plan. We emphasize these nutritious foods.

Eating some food from each of the four corners of the diet every day makes it easy to make sure you're eating a variety of foods and getting a balance of nutrients instead of filling up on meat alone. By following the Four Corners Diet, you'll not only lose weight, you'll improve your overall health at the same time.

And it doesn't have to be difficult: "There is such a variety of foods, and you never feel hungry," said Lisa K., who went from a size 16–18 to a size 8–10 and has kept the weight off for two years.

BENEFITS OF CORNER 1: LOW-CARB EATING

IF YOU ARE very overweight, you most certainly also have something called hyperinsulinemia. What's that? It means you have high levels of the hormone insulin in your blood. You have a chronic disease.

Yes, we said disease. You have a chronic illness, and unless you face that fact, you're not going to get well (slim). You have tried treating the symptoms (your weight problem), but until you treat your underlying disease, you're not going to have permanent results.

What is insulin? It's the hormone your pancreas produces to help move the sugar in your blood into the muscles, where the sugar can be burned for energy. For some reason no one really understands yet, when you're overweight, your body develops something called insulin resistance, which means your muscles resist the actions of insulin. You need to produce a lot more insulin to do the job. The result is hyperinsulinemia, or high levels of insulin in the blood. High insulin levels further increase the insulin resistance. This means your pancreas produces yet more insulin. You're caught in a vicious circle that can—if you have the genetic predisposition—burn out your pancreas and lead to diabetes. High insulin levels have also been associated with increased rates of heart disease.

Eating carbohydrates is what makes insulin levels increase. In thin people without insulin resistance, this is not a problem. They can eat carbohydrates, their blood sugar goes up a little bit, their pancreas produces a little insulin, the sugar resulting from the carbohydrates they ate gets carried into their cells and burned for energy, and the pancreas stops producing insulin. This is the way the body is supposed to work.

Unfortunately, in some people things don't work this way. You eat carbohydrates and because of your insulin resistance, your pancreas has to produce a lot of insulin to carry the glucose into your cells. Even with this extra insulin, it may take a long time for your glucose levels to return to normal.

Insulin also tells fat cells to store fat and to resist releasing any fat that's already stored. And, sad to say, the fat cells can be less insulin resistant

NET CARBOHYDRATE GRAMS

Net carbohydrate means the carbohydrates remaining aft_ tract the indigestible fiber from the total carbohydrate con_ food (fiber is a carbohydrate, but humans can't digest it). You can eat as much fiber as you want, and in fact, the more the better. So remember: *Fiber doesn't count.*

Net carbs = Total carbs – Fiber

However, a word of warning. The above applies to nutrition labels on American foods. In the United Kingdom, Europe, and Australia, the fiber has already been subtracted, and the label reports the net carbs. For example, let's say a piece of crispbread from Norway contains 4 grams of fiber and 5 grams of other carbohydrates.

If this product were made in America, the label would report:

Carbohydrate: 9 grams
Fiber: 4 grams

and you would subtract 4 from 9 to get the 5 grams of net carbs in the product.

But the label on the product from Europe would report:

Carbohydrate: 5 grams
Fiber: 4 grams

and you would *not* subtract the fiber from the carbohydrate. If you did, you would think you were eating less carbohydrate than you actually were.

Canada, Africa, and Asia usually follow the American system. Oceania usually follows the European system. But regulations in individual countries may change, so if you eat a lot of these foods, try to find out what system they're using.

than the cells in the muscles. This means that if normal insulin levels—those you'd find in a thin person—tell the fat cells to "store fat," the high insulin levels found in someone with insulin resistance tell the fat cells to **"STORE FAT!"** And because insulin levels are high for a longer period

. time than normal, the fat-storing message persists for a longer time and you'll store more fat than normal. No wonder you have a problem.

Insulin also speeds up the process with which the liver converts any extra glucose from your food into fat. In overweight people, this process is speeded up even more than in thin people.

Although the amount of fat produced by this process after each meal may be relatively small (most of the extra glucose is stored in the liver in a storage compound called glycogen), a little bit at each meal adds up. A few ounces a day will turn into pounds every year. And the insulin tells the body to store all that fat in the fat cells.

Now you should see why low-fat, high-carbohydrate diets didn't work for you. Eating carbohydrates is sabotaging everything you're trying to accomplish. If you want to lose weight and keep it off, *you must be willing to face your problem and give up all high-carbohydrate foods.*

Don't worry. It's not as bad as it sounds. We didn't say you have to give up *all* carbohydrate foods. Just those with high carbohydrate loads, above 3 or 4 *net carbohydrate grams* per serving (see box on page 15).

Fiber doesn't count. Most vegetables contain carbohydrates, but except in very starchy vegetables like potatoes and corn, a lot of that carbohydrate is in the form of fiber, which you can subtract from the total.

What you need to avoid are starches and sugars. For you these are poison. You'll have to stay away from any processed cereal grains and flours, as well conventional breads, cereals, cookies, or pastas. You'll have to avoid starchy vegetables like corn, peas, potatoes, beans, and lentils. Also any sugars such as candies, sweets, sodas, puddings, milk, and nearly all fruit.

These are the foods that keep your fat cells from giving up their fat.

Right now you may be thinking, "I couldn't do this." That's wrong. Very wrong. We've done it. Hundreds of people have done it. You can do it, too. You must do it, because it can be your salvation.

When you start the diet, your cravings for these high-carbohydrate foods won't last more than three or four days. From then on, you won't crave them. That doesn't mean you won't miss them. Of course you will. You're human. But you won't crave them, so you'll have the willpower to resist them.

When you follow the Four Corners Diet, not only your cravings but also your hunger pangs will decrease. Eating a lot of carbohydrate foods—especially the highly processed carbohydrate foods that snack manufacturers love to sell us—makes your blood sugar level go up a lot, so your body produces a lot of insulin to bring your blood sugar level back down again.

Sometimes you produce *too much* insulin, and then your blood sugar goes *too low* a few hours after you eat. Low blood sugar makes you hungry. Ravenously hungry. So you eat more carbohydrate snacks, which drives your blood sugar too high again, and then more insulin makes it go too low again. You're on a constant blood sugar roller coaster.

Avoiding these high-carbohydrate foods will keep your blood sugar levels on an even keel, and your hunger will abate. Without this unnatural blood sugar roller coaster and unnatural hunger, your body should tell you how much to eat to maintain a healthy weight, and you should be able to listen to your body's messages.

What are these messages? No one knows for sure. There are many hormonal signals given off by fat tissue and gut tissue—and new ones are discovered every year—that tell the brain to increase or decrease your appetite to maintain a healthy weight. In a natural environment, you probably wouldn't want to make an effort to hunt for food if you weren't really hungry. Lions don't. But the body's signals can be blunted by the unnatural conditions of modern living. We don't have to hunt for food. We are surrounded by it. We do a lot of social eating.

If you're not ravenously hungry, it's a lot easier to resist the siren's song of social eating, which usually focuses on high-carbohydrate treats. The benefits of feeling better and losing weight will outweigh any remaining pangs of longing for your old carby friends.

BENEFITS OF CORNER 2: MONOUNSATURATED FAT

AS MENTIONED IN Chapter 2, eating a lot of saturated fat affects your weight, increases your insulin resistance, and raises your cholesterol levels. This can result in hypertension, diabetes, and heart disease. You should be aware that all the studies showing a relation between saturated fat and these problems have been done with diets that also contained a lot of carbohydrates. To date, we have not found a single study showing the effects of a reasonable amount of saturated fat on people eating a diet low in carbohydrates.

Nevertheless, we decided to take a conservative approach and, for the present at least, recommend that you limit your consumption of saturated fat and focus on monounsaturated fat instead.

> ## TYPES OF FAT
>
> **Fats are made** up of fatty acids and glycerin. It's the fatty acid content of a fat that determines what kind of fat we call it. Saturated fats—for example, animal fats such as butter, lard, and beef tallow, and tropical fats such as coconut oil—are solid at room temperature. Unsaturated fats—for example olive oil, soybean oil, corn oil, peanut oil—are liquid at room temperature.
>
> Note that no fats contain only one kind of fatty acid or another. We simply label them according to their major constituent. Even lard contains a lot of unsaturated fatty acids. Olive oil contains some saturated fatty acids. The more unsaturated fatty acids there are in a particular fat, the less solid it is. For example, lamb fat contains a lot of saturated fatty acids and may harden on your plate at room temperature. Chicken fat contains more unsaturated fatty acids and is much more liquid at room temperature than beef fat.

On a traditional diet that includes both fat and carbohydrates, saturated fat tends to increase your cholesterol levels more than the amount of cholesterol you eat in your food. But when people go on a very low-carbohydrate diet, about 70 percent usually see their cholesterol levels decrease, *even when they eat a lot of saturated fat.*

Unfortunately, about 30 percent of people on very low-carbohydrate diets do *not* see their cholesterol levels decrease when they eat a lot of saturated fat. They may even find that their cholesterol levels go up. However, a high consumption of monounsaturated fat can counter this effect. Substituting monounsaturated fat for saturated fat may also reduce insulin resistance, and insulin resistance which can lead to type 2 diabetes. Finally, monounsaturated fat may provide some degree of protection against some cancers.

Hence, even if you're in the lucky group that sees cholesterol levels fall on a low-carb diet that includes a lot of saturated fat, you'll be better off focusing on monounsaturated fat instead.

■

BENEFITS OF CORNER 3:
FIBER

FIBER IS A form of carbohydrate that humans can't digest. This means it has very few calories. We say "very few" instead of "zero" because although you can't digest the fiber with human enzymes, bacteria in your colon can digest many types of fiber, and you can obtain some calories from the products of that digestion.

You may have noticed the effects of another product of the bacteria: gas. High-fiber foods sometimes make you produce a lot of gas (the well-known bean effect).

Nevertheless, fiber has many benefits. There are two different types of fiber: soluble fiber and insoluble fiber. As you might expect, soluble fiber is soluble in water. It forms a gel, like gelatin dessert. Insoluble fiber, like sawdust, does not dissolve in water. Both types of fiber are beneficial to your health.

One benefit is that fiber holds water. This increases the bulk of stools and reduces constipation. This is how many over-the-counter constipation fixers, such as those containing psyllium, work. Because low-carb diets without sufficient vegetables and fiber tend to produce constipation, this is an important part of this diet.

A second benefit is that soluble fiber binds to compounds like cholesterol, so more of the cholesterol in your system is excreted in the stool. The result is lower cholesterol levels. Soluble fiber also slows down the rate at which your stomach empties. This means that whatever small amounts of carbohydrates are in your diet are released into the intestine more slowly and steadily, so your blood sugar levels won't increase as fast and then possibly plummet too fast because of oversecretion of insulin. This is a special benefit to people with carbohydrate disturbances such as diabetes or low blood sugar problems.

Fiber may also reduce the risks of disease by binding carcinogens and environmental toxins so they are not absorbed.

Fiber is found in vegetables, and the less starchy the vegetable, the greater the proportion of healthy fiber. Fruits and whole grains also contain a lot of fiber. Unfortunately, these also contain a lot of carbohydrates. However, both insoluble fiber (for example, bran) and soluble fiber (for example, psyllium and guar gum) can be isolated from grains and other foods and added to foods to increase their fiber content.

DISSOLVING GUMS

Soluble fibers like psyllium husks or powder and guar gum or xanthan make a healthy addition to your diet. This is especially true if you have type 2 diabetes and want to make sure your stomach empties slowly, so your sluggish pancreas will be able to produce enough insulin to cover the carbohydrate foods you eat.

(Note: If you have the diabetic complication gastroparesis, slowing down the emptying of your stomach even further is not a good idea, and you should not add a lot of soluble fiber to your diet without checking first with your doctor.)

When using these gums, remember that a little bit goes a long way. And sometimes they can cause problems. If you use too much gum without enough water, they can form sticky globs that won't dissolve no matter what you do. In fact, if you eat a lot of gums without sufficient water, they can form globs in your intestine that can cause blockage. So remember to dissolve them in plenty of liquid.

The best way to dissolve these gums is to sprinkle a tiny bit on top of the liquid and stir. Wait a bit, and if it doesn't get thick enough, add a little more. Unless you're following a recipe that gives the amount to use, add a little at a time until the product reaches the thickness you want. Sometimes they get thicker with standing.

Guar especially is soluble in both cold and hot water. What this means is that you shouldn't use the trick you've probably learned to dissolve cornstarch. Cornstarch isn't soluble in cold water. What you usually do is *suspend* it in cold water. Then you heat it to get it to dissolve and form a gel. If you try this trick with gums, you'll probably end up with a thick glob that won't dissolve even when you heat it.

BENEFITS OF CORNER 4:
PHARMAFOODS

WE'RE USING THE term *pharmafoods* to mean foods that have health benefits beyond their content of vitamins and minerals. These include the probiotic foods—yogurt, kefir, buttermilk, and other fermented foods such as raw sauerkraut—and the other pharmafoods that contain disease-preventing and disease-fighting phytochemicals.

Probiotic Foods

A bacterium called *Lactobacillus* and other similar bacteria convert milk into buttermilk, yogurt, and kefir. These bacteria are also normally present in the human bowels and in the human female vagina and help to keep these organs healthy. Unfortunately, our modern high-carbohydrate diet and the use of antibiotics can disrupt the normal colonization by these lactic acid bacteria and lead to gastrointestinal complaints and yeast infections. A steady intake of lactic acid bacteria helps to maintain a healthy bowel and vagina. Hence we recommend eating at least 1 cup of live-culture fermented milk products every day. The milk-fermenting bacteria have also been found to stimulate the immune system, in addition to forming a great deal of bulk so you will have well-formed, nonconstipating stools.

If you think you can't eat milk products because you're lactose intolerant (lactose is the name of the natural sugar found in milk), don't worry. The bacteria convert most of the lactose in the milk into lactic acid, which your body can digest.

The lactic acid produced by the bacteria is a natural antimicrobial and may protect you somewhat from *Shigella* and *Salmonella* poisoning. Indeed, daily consumption of yogurt while traveling may protect you from traveler's diarrhea. Yogurt may also help with antibiotic-associated diarrhea. Because the bacteria in these fermented milk products break down the milk sugar, yogurt won't raise your blood sugar levels as much as milk, a great benefit to those with diabetes.

Research has shown that probiotics may help degrade cholesterol. Animal research has shown that probiotics enhance T-cell immunity. And finally, milk products are a good source of calcium. You won't be drinking milk on this diet, so eating enough yogurt to supply calcium is important.

Other Pharmafoods

Many vegetables and fruits are healthy. But some are healthier than others. These foods, which we have put into the pharmafoods category, supply natural sources of antioxidants and other phytochemicals as well as minerals, trace elements, and vitamins.

Antioxidants are important because they help reduce the risk of injury to blood vessels, lowering your risk of heart disease and stroke. They also help reduce your risk of cancer. Antioxidants include the vitamins A, C, and E, beta carotene, lycopene, lutein, flavonoids, lipoic acid, and polyphenols.

Examples of foods that are good low-carbohydrate sources of antioxidants include greens, kale, spinach, romaine lettuce, fennel, all types of squash, broccoli, Brussels sprouts, cauliflower, nuts, edible seeds, avocados, celery, onions, leeks, soybeans, peppers, cabbage, watermelon, cantaloupe, strawberries, kiwis, and blueberries. Beverages include tea, coffee, and red wine.

The pharmafoods also contain cancer-inhibiting ingredients. Isothiocyanates, found in cruciferous vegetables (like broccoli, cauliflower, and Brussels sprouts) have been shown to help inhibit cancer growth.

The lycopenes in tomatoes have been shown to protect against prostate cancer, especially when the tomatoes are cooked.

Phytoestrogens, which inhibit estrogen production, and indoles, which convert estrogen into a more harmless hormone, may inhibit tumors whose growth is promoted by natural estrogen production. Cruciferous vegetables and soybeans contain these substances.

Allicin, a substance found in garlic, leeks, onions, and scallions, is an additional chemical that has been associated with a reduction in blood pressure and in cholesterol. These same foods also contain sulfur-allyl cysteine, which, along with other sulfur compounds, has been associated with cancer prevention, by blocking effects of carcinogens in the gastrointestinal tract.

We expect this corner to grow in the future as research demonstrates further beneficial properties of more foods.

This has been a brief outline of the benefits of the Four Corners Diet. If you'd like to read more on the science of the diet, you can skip to Chapter 13. If you're ready to start, the next chapter will get you going.

▶ IF YOU HAVE DIABETES

IF YOU HAVE type 2 diabetes, you're probably overweight and you'd undoubtedly like to lose some of that weight. Losing weight will reduce your insulin resistance, and because insulin resistance is the cause of type 2 diabetes (by definition), losing weight can increase your control of the disease.

This diet will help you lose weight. However, you should be aware that there is no guarantee that weight loss alone will control your type 2 diabetes. The effect of weight loss on blood glucose control depends in part on how far your diabetes has progressed.

If you were diagnosed in the early stages, weight loss may in fact reverse the condition and—as long as you keep the weight off—allow you to stay free of diabetes medications for a long time. However, if you weren't diagnosed until later in this progressive disease, weight loss alone may not have much effect on your blood sugar control. Most people who see an effect of weight loss on blood sugar see it when they've lost about ten pounds. If you see no effect at this point, you probably won't see any even if you lose a lot more.

But this diet does more than help you lose weight. A diet that is low in carbohydrate and high in fiber will reduce your blood sugar levels almost immediately, even before you have lost any weight. The reason is simple. Carbohydrates make your blood sugar go up. When you stop eating huge amounts of carbohydrates, your blood sugar levels will stay lower.

The fiber in the diet will also slow down the rate at which your stomach empties. The small amounts of carbohydrates in the vegetables you eat will be released slowly, so your ailing pancreas can deal with them better.

When you have type 2 diabetes, getting enough antioxidants is important, because high blood sugar levels are associated with oxidative damage, and people with type 2 diabetes tend to be low in antioxidants.

Finally, if you have diabetes, you're in this for the long haul: at the present time diabetes is not curable. However, diabetes *can* be controlled, and a healthy diet plays a large part in that control. You need a diet that is healthy and varied enough that you can stick with it for the rest of your life. The Four Corners Diet should fill the bill.

FOUR

Phase 1: Getting Started

BEFORE YOU START

YOU MAY START this diet now if you are healthy. But first you should see your doctor and have some lab tests done. Then you can have the tests repeated in eight to twelve weeks to see what kind of progress you're making.

It is especially important to see your doctor before making any drastic change in your diet if you have any kind of medical condition or have a strong family history of cardiac disease, diabetes, or hypertension, especially if you're on medication, because diet and weight loss can affect blood pressure and blood sugar levels, and you may need to reduce your medications.

Ask your physician or health clinic for a full lipid profile and have them measure your glucose and creatinine levels. Although it is not commonly ordered, your doctor may also want to measure your fasting insulin level. The various tests are described in more detail in Chapter 13.

You should also measure your body mass index, usually referred to as BMI. The formal definition of BMI is

$$BMI = WEIGHT\ IN\ KILOGRAMS \div (HEIGHT\ IN\ METERS)^2$$

But don't worry. You don't need to do all those conversions. Just measure your weight in pounds and your height in inches and use the numbers in Table 4.1. You can also find BMI calculators on various Web sites. Just type "body mass index" into your favorite search engine. You fill in the numbers and the computer does an exact calculation.

TABLE 4.1
Find Your Body Mass Index

❖

IF YOUR HEIGHT OR WEIGHT FALLS BETWEEN TWO NUMBERS, ESTIMATE YOUR BMI BY AVERAGING.												
	4'10"	5'0"	5'2"	5'4"	5'6"	5'8"	5'10"	6'0"	6'2"	6'4"	6'6"	6'8"
95	19.9	18.6	17.4	16.4	15.4	14.5						
100	21.0	19.6	18.4	17.2	16.2	15.3	14.4					
105	22.0	20.6	19.3	18.1	17.0	16.0	15.1	14.3				
110	23.1	21.6	20.2	18.9	17.8	16.8	15.8	15.0	14.2			
115	24.1	22.5	21.1	19.8	18.6	17.5	16.6	15.7	14.8	14.0		
120	25.2	23.5	22.0	20.7	19.4	18.3	17.3	16.3	15.5	14.7		
125	26.2	24.5	22.9	21.5	20.2	19.1	18.0	17.0	16.1	15.3	14.5	
130	27.3	25.5	23.9	22.4	21.1	19.8	18.7	17.7	16.8	15.9	15.1	14.3
135	28.3	26.5	24.8	23.3	21.9	20.6	19.4	18.4	17.4	16.5	15.7	14.9
140	29.4	27.4	25.7	24.1	22.7	21.4	20.2	19.1	18.0	17.1	16.2	15.4
145	30.4	28.4	26.6	25.0	23.5	22.1	20.9	19.7	18.7	17.7	16.8	16.0
150	31.5	29.4	27.5	25.8	24.3	22.9	21.6	20.4	19.3	18.3	17.4	16.5
155	32.5	30.4	28.5	26.7	25.1	23.7	22.3	21.1	20.0	18.9	18.0	17.1
160	33.6	31.4	29.4	27.6	25.9	24.4	23.0	21.8	20.6	19.5	18.6	17.6
165	34.6	32.3	30.3	28.4	26.7	25.2	23.8	22.5	21.3	20.2	19.1	18.2
170	35.7	33.3	31.2	29.3	27.5	25.9	24.5	23.1	21.9	20.8	19.7	18.7
175	36.7	34.3	32.1	30.1	28.3	26.7	25.2	23.8	22.5	21.4	20.3	19.3
180	37.8	35.3	33.0	31.0	29.2	27.5	25.9	24.5	23.2	22.0	20.9	19.8
185	38.8	36.3	34.0	31.9	30.0	28.2	26.6	25.2	23.8	22.6	21.5	20.4
190	39.9	37.2	34.9	32.7	30.8	29.0	27.4	25.9	24.5	23.2	22.0	20.9
195	40.9	38.2	35.8	33.6	31.6	29.8	28.1	26.5	25.1	23.8	22.6	21.5

YOUR WEIGHT IN POUNDS

IF YOUR HEIGHT OR WEIGHT FALLS BETWEEN TWO NUMBERS, ESTIMATE YOUR BMI BY AVERAGING.												
	4'10"	5'0"	5'2"	5'4"	5'6"	5'8"	5'10"	6'0"	6'2"	6'4"	6'6"	6'8"
200	42.0	39.2	36.7	34.5	32.4	30.5	28.8	27.2	25.8	24.4	23.2	22.1
205	43.0	40.2	37.6	35.3	33.2	31.3	29.5	27.9	26.4	25.0	23.8	22.6
210	44.0	41.2	38.5	36.2	34.0	32.0	30.2	28.6	27.1	25.7	24.4	23.2
215	45.1	42.1	39.5	37.0	34.8	32.8	31.0	29.3	27.7	26.3	24.9	23.7
220	46.1	43.1	40.4	37.9	35.6	33.6	31.7	29.9	28.3	26.9	25.5	24.3
225	47.2	44.1	41.3	38.8	36.4	34.3	32.4	30.6	29.0	27.5	26.1	24.8
230	48.2	45.1	42.2	39.6	37.3	35.1	33.1	31.3	29.6	28.1	26.7	25.4
235	49.3	46.1	43.1	40.5	38.1	35.9	33.8	32.0	30.3	28.7	27.3	25.9
240	50.3	47.0	44.1	41.3	38.9	36.6	34.6	32.7	30.9	29.3	27.8	26.5
245	51.4	48.0	45.0	42.2	39.7	37.4	35.3	33.3	31.6	29.9	28.4	27.0
250	52.4	49.0	45.9	43.1	40.5	38.1	36.0	34.0	32.2	30.5	29.0	27.6
255	53.5	50.0	46.8	43.9	41.3	38.9	36.7	34.7	32.9	31.2	29.6	28.1
260	54.5	51.0	47.7	44.8	42.1	39.7	37.4	35.4	33.5	31.8	30.2	28.7
265	55.6	51.9	48.6	45.7	42.9	40.4	38.2	36.1	34.1	32.4	30.7	29.2
270	56.6	52.9	49.6	46.5	43.7	41.2	38.9	36.8	34.8	33.0	31.3	29.8

(YOUR WEIGHT IN POUNDS — left axis)

Find your weight at the left of the table and go across that row until you're in the column that represents your height. That's your BMI. If your height falls within two points on the table, average the results from the two points. For example, if you're five feet seven inches and weigh 170 pounds, average 27.5 (for five feet six inches) and 25.9 (for five feet eight inches), for a BMI of 26.7. You can do the same if your weight falls between two points on the left.

The World Health Organization has defined desired BMIs as 25 or less. If your BMI is 25 to 30, you are considered overweight. If your BMI is more than 30, you are considered obese. For someone five feet eight inches tall, this would be about two hundred pounds.

If you have a BMI of 25 or higher (boldface on table), you will see the greatest weight loss on the Four Corners Diet. If your BMI is less than 25, you're within the normal range, even if you'd like to lose a few pounds, and you probably won't lose much weight. But you certainly will be a lot healthier. The diet should also help you if you have problems with low blood sugar, high triglycerides, hyperinsulinemia, prediabetes, or diabetes, even if you don't need to lose a lot of weight.

While you're measuring your BMI, record a few more measurements so you can see your progress as you go along. Get out a tape measure and measure your waist at the belly button and your hips at their widest part. Write these measurements down and put them away somewhere. We want you to make the same measurements in twelve weeks and compare them with your starting measurements. You'll get a pleasant surprise.

CONCENTRATE ON NET CARBOHYDRATE LOAD

IN THIS FIRST phase of the diet, which lasts only three days, you're going to greatly reduce the amount of carbohydrates in your diet. Your goal will be 50 grams of *net* carbohydrates a day, with no more than 12 to 15 grams of *net* carbohydrates at any one meal.

Reducing your carbohydrate intake like this will give your body a chance to gear up for burning fat instead of carbohydrate for its energy needs. The little furnaces in your cells called mitochondria are where the fat is burned. We need to send a loud and clear message to these little fat-burning machines that they are going to have to increase production. All leave has been canceled. This message will be sent by greatly reducing the amount of carbohydrate in your diet.

What is carbohydrate? Carbohydrate means starches and sugars: breads; cereals; cookies; pastas; starchy vegetables like corn, peas, potatoes, beans, and lentils; and sugars such as candies, sweets, sodas, puddings, milk, and nearly all fruit.

We'll bet that your diet today consists primarily of low-fiber carbohydrate foods. Something like this: Bagel or cereal, coffee, and juice for breakfast. Followed by a "little piece" of coffee cake and coffee at ten o'clock break. Burger, fries, and a soda around noon, followed by a candy bar or cookies or chips or pretzels and soda in the afternoon or on the way home in the car or on the train, followed by a couple of chips or cookies while making dinner, which includes pasta, potato, or rice and a little dessert. And maybe a cookie before bed. With a few variations, maybe soup and salad with bread for lunch, we'll bet this is pretty close to what you've been eating when you're not on a grapefruit or a cabbage diet.

Net carbohydrate (see box on page 15) means the carbohydrates remaining after you subtract the indigestible fiber from the total carbohydrate content of the food (remember, fiber is a carbohydrate, but humans can't digest it). You can eat as much fiber as you want; your goal should be 25 to 30 grams. But don't start with a lot of fiber right away. Work up to it slowly.

During Phase 1 of the diet, we want you to concentrate solely on the net carbohydrate content of the foods you eat. This is probably the most difficult part of the diet. But we know you're motivated and you can do it.

To do this, you will need to determine the net carbohydrate content of all the foods you eat. You can find the carbohydrate contents of many foods in nutrition books, in small carbohydrate counters, in nutritional software programs, on Internet nutrition sites (type "carbohydrate counter" or "nutrition analysis" into your favorite search engine), and on the nutrition labels of foods. To get you started, Table 4.2 gives the net carbohydrate content of some common foods (for now, don't worry about the monounsaturated fat content). You can copy this short list and carry it with you wherever you go.

TABLE 4.2
Net Carbohydrate and Monounsaturated Content of Food
Net carbs = Total carbs – Fiber

FOOD	GRAMS/CUP	NET CARBS	% MONO
Asparagus, raw	134	3.2	
Avocado, raw, California	230	4.6	64.6
Avocado, raw, Florida	230	13.8	55.1
Bamboo shoots	131	2.4	
Beans, snap, green, canned solids	135	3.5	
Beef franks (5 in long x $^3/_4$ in diameter)	45 g each	1.8	47.7
Beef, ground, lean (< 21% fat)		0	42.9
Beef tenderloin, lean, trimmed		0	37.7
Beef round, tip, all fat trimmed		0	40.9
Broccoli, raw, chopped	88	2.7	
Brussels sprouts	1 g each	1	
Cabbage (Chinese bok choy)	170	0.3	
Cabbage, raw (shredded)	70	2.2	
Carrots (baby raw)	1 g each	0.8	
Cauliflower, raw pieces	100	4	
Celery, raw	120	2.4	
Cheese, cottage, uncreamed	145	2.7	26.2
Cheese, cottage, creamed	220	5.9	28.8
Cheese, cottage, 1% fat	226	6.1	28.4
Cheese, brie (melted)	240	1.2	28.6
Cheese, cheddar (diced)	132	1.7	28.4
Cheese, Colby (diced)	132	3.4	28.9
Cheese, cream	232	6.3	28.2
Cheese, feta (crumbled)	150	6.2	21.7
Cheese, mozzarella, part skim	112	3.1	28.3
Cheese, mozzarella, whole milk	112	2.5	30.1

Phase 1: Getting Started

FOOD	GRAMS/CUP	NET CARBS	% MONO
Cheese, Parmesan, grated	100	3.7	29.0
Cheese, ricotta, whole milk	246	7.4	27.7
Cheese, Swiss (diced)	132	4.5	26.5
Chicken breast, with skin	145	0	40.9
Chicken leg	167	0	40.5
Chives, raw, chopped	1 g/teaspoon	1.9	
Coffee, brewed with tap water	237	0.9	
Cranberries, raw, chopped	110	9.4	
Cream, half-and-half	242	10.4	28.9
Cream, heavy whipping	238	6.7	28.9
Cream, sour, cultured	230	9.9	28.6
Cress, garden, raw	50	2.2	
Cucumber with peel, raw	104	2	
Dandelion greens, raw	55	3.1	
Egg, hard-boiled, whole (chopped)	136	1.5	38.5
Egg, whole, raw, large	50 g each	1.2	
Eggplant, raw, cubed	82	3	
Endive, raw	50	0.2	
Fish, gefilte, sweet	42 g/piece	3	48.2
Fish, herring, pickled	140	13.4	66.1
Frankfurter, beef, each	approx. 50 g	1.8	
Ginger root, raw	2 g/teaspoon	13	
Gooseberries, raw	150	8.9	
Grapefruit, raw	100	6.9	
Heart of palms, canned	146	3.2	
Kohlrabi, raw	135	3.8	
Kiwis, store-bought	91 g each	10.5	
Kale, raw	67	5.4	
Leeks, lower portion, raw	89	11.0	
Lettuce, cos or romaine, raw	56	0.4	
Lettuce, iceberg, raw	55	0.4	
Melon, cantaloupe	177	13.5	
Melon, casaba	170	9.2	
Melon, honeydew	177	15	
Melon, watermelon	154	10.5	
Mung beans, sprouted, raw	104	4.3	
Mushrooms, raw	70	2.5	
Nuts, almonds, roasted, blanched	142	9.7	65.5

FOOD	GRAMS/CUP	NET CARB	% MONO
Nuts, Brazil, dried, unblanched	140	10.4	34.8
Nuts, coconut meat, desiccated unsweetened	8.1	4.3	
Nuts, coconut meat, raw, shredded	80	5	4.2
Nuts, hazelnuts, dried, chopped	115	10.6	78.4
Nuts, macadamia, oil roasted with salt	134	4.8	78.9
Nuts, pecans, oil roasted with salt	110	10.3	62.4
Okra, raw	100	4.4	
Onions, raw	160	10.9	
Onions, spring, raw, chopped	100	4.7	
Papaya, raw, cubed	140	11.2	
Parsley, raw	60	1.8	
Peanuts, Spanish, raw	146	9.2	44.7
Peanut butter, smooth, with salt	258	38.2	47.0
Peppers, sweet, green, raw	149	6.9	
Peppers, sweet, red, raw	149	6.6	
Peppers, sweet, yellow, raw	149	8.0	
Pickles, cucumber, sour	155	1.6	
Pickles, cucumber, dill	143	4.2	
Plums, raw	66	7.6	
Prickly pears, raw	149	8.9	
Potato skins, raw	100	9.9	
Pumpkin, canned	245	12.7	
Pumpkin, raw, cubed	116	7	
Radicchio, raw	40	1.4	
Radishes, white icicle, raw	100	1.2	
Radishes, raw	116	2.3	
Raspberries, raw	123	5.9	
Rhubarb, raw	122	3.3	
Rutabaga, raw	140	7.8	
Salami, cooked beef, slice	23	0.6	44.8
Salmon, red, canned	369/1-lb can	0	38.4
Sardines, in tomato sauce, drained	89	0	45.8
Sauerkraut, canned, undrained	142	2.6	
Soy flour, full-fat	84	20.7	21.8
Spinach, raw	30	0.2	
Squash, summer, sliced, raw	113	2.8	
Squash, winter, raw, all varieties	116	8.5	
Squash, spaghetti, raw	101	6.5	

FOOD	GRAMS/CUP		
Strawberries, raw	152		
Tofu, raw, firm	126		
Tomatillos, raw, diced	132		
Tomatoes, raw, red, ripe	180		
Tuna, white, canned, drained	172		
Turnips, raw, cubed	130		
Veggie burgers (Morningstar)	110	1.5	35.6
Water chestnuts, Chinese, canned	140	13.9	
Wheat bran, crude	58	12.6	41.7
Yogurt, plain, 8 g protein/8 ounces	245	approx. 4	27.7

Net carbs are per cup unless otherwise indicated.

If this seems too complicated at first, we've provided a set of menus for the first seven days of the diet. You don't have to follow these menus to succeed on the diet. But they're there in case you don't want to calculate carb counts by yourself.

■

EAT AS MUCH AS YOU LIKE

THIS DIET DOES not restrict the number of calories you consume. It restricts only the amount of carbohydrate. As long as you don't eat more than 12 to 15 grams of net carbs per meal and 50 grams of net carbs per day, you can eat as much food as you need to satisfy your hunger.

During Phase 1, you can eat any of the foods listed in Table 4.3. *Do not eat anything that is not listed in this table, not even a taste.* This is very important. If you want this diet to work for you, you must start out with this three-day regimen. We explain why in Chapter 13. Note that you're not allowed any fruit in Phase 1. But after three days, small amounts of fruit can be added back into your diet.

TABLE 4.3
Foods Allowed on First Three Days of the Four Corners Diet
❖

MEATS/FISH/EGGS/NUTS	DAIRY	VEGETABLES	OTHER
Any meat, trimmed of all excess fat and unbreaded	Kefir, yogurt, or buttermilk, plain, unsweetened, or	Cucumbers, lettuce, greens, spinach, olives,	Mayonnaise, sugar-free, condiments, sour pickles,
Any fish or shellfish, unbreaded	sweetened by you	broccoli, cauliflower,	sugar-free gelatin,
Canned fish in oil	with artificial	mushrooms, celery,	spices, salt, pepper, no-
Eggs	sweeteners	Chinese vegetables	calorie sweeteners
All nuts, except pistachios and cashews	Cheeses, unsweetened:	(bean sprouts, bok choy,	
Edible seeds (sunflower kernels, pumpkin seeds)	cheddar, Swiss,	bamboo shoots, greens),	
	mozzarella, ricotta,	zucchini, onions, asparagus,	
	cream	cabbage, sauerkraut	
	Real cream, unsweetened		

To cook your protein foods, you can broil, bake, grill, boil, or pan-fry them in olive or canola oil. Use oil and vinegar or full-fat unsweetened salad dressings. Olive oil dressings are best, but for now, focus just on the carb counts. *Check the labels of all the packaged foods you buy to make sure they're not high in carbohydrate.*

Drink diet soda, coffee, tea, water, plain or artificially sweetened kefir, or buttermilk. No other milk of any type is allowed. Refrain from any alcohol for these first three days.

Eat three meals a day, and snack whenever you feel like it. *Don't skip any meals.* Use cheese cubes, string cheese, tuna, or chicken drumsticks or wings (roasted, seasoned with salt and pepper, dipped in no-carb condiments) for snacks.

Because you're just starting and this is a transition-phase diet, take one multivitamin-and-mineral supplement a day.

Remember, don't count calories. We mean it. *Do not count calories or fat during these first three days.* You should concentrate on one goal alone during these first three days: getting the carbohydrates out of your daily diet.

Table 4.4 provides sample menus. You do not need to follow these menus exactly. You can eat the foods indicated, but eat less if you're full with less or eat more of the noncarby foods if you're still hungry.

TABLE 4.4.
Seven Days of Menus

◼ DAY 1 ◼

	CARBS, GRAMS	FIBER, GRAMS	NET CARBS
BREAKFAST			
2 eggs with 1 teaspoon butter	1	0	1
3 large slices bacon (or sausage)	0	0	0
Breakfast TOTAL*	**1**	**0**	**1**
LUNCH			
6 ounces canned tuna in oil	0	0	0
2 cups mixed salad greens with:	3	1	2
5 large ripe olives	1	1	0
lemon and oil dressing (2 teaspoons lemon juice			
and 2 teaspoons olive oil) (or mayonnaise)	1	0	1
1 large sour pickle	3	2	1
Lunch TOTAL*	**8**	**3**	**5**
DINNER			
8 ounces roast chicken (or turkey) with skin	0	0	0
1 cup cauliflower, mashed	5	3	2
1 cup broccoli	8	5	3
2 cups mixed salad greens with:	3	1	2
vinegar and oil dressing (2 teaspoons vinegar			
and 2 teaspoons olive oil)	0	0	0
1 cup (or more or less) sugar-free gelatin dessert with:	2	0	2
1 tablespoon whipped cream	0	0	0
Dinner TOTAL*	**18**	**9**	**9**
SNACKS			
2 ounces cheddar cheese (or other hard cheese)	1	0	1
TOTAL FOR DAY*	**28**	**12**	**16**

▦ DAY 2 ▦

	CARBS, GRAMS	FIBER, GRAMS	NET CARBS
BREAKFAST			
Ham and cheese omelet made with:			
2 eggs	1	0	1
1 ounce cheddar cheese	0	0	0
2 ounces ham	0	0	0
1 teaspoon butter and 1 teaspoon olive oil for frying	0	0	0
Breakfast TOTAL*	**2**	**0**	**2**
LUNCH			
Chef's salad made with:			
2 cups iceberg lettuce	2	2	0
1 ounce Swiss cheese	1	0	1
2 hard-boiled eggs	1	0	1
2 ounces turkey breast	0	0	0
5 black olives, chopped	1	1	0
1 tablespoon ranch dressing (or oil and vinegar)	1	0	1
Lunch TOTAL*	**7**	**3**	**4**
DINNER			
6 ounces roast pork	0	0	0
1 cup green beans	10	4	6
½ cup sauerkraut	5	3	2
1 cup cucumbers with 2 tablespoons sour cream (or oil and vinegar)	4	1	3
Diet chocolate fudge (or root beer) soda with 1 ounce (2 tablespoons) heavy cream and ice	0	0	0
Dinner TOTAL*	**20**	**8**	**12**
SNACKS			
2 ounces cheddar cheese (or other hard cheese)	1	0	1
TOTAL FOR DAY*	**29**	**10**	**19**

▦ DAY 3 ▦

	CARBS, GRAMS	FIBER, GRAMS	NET CARBS
BREAKFAST			
4 ounces smoked salmon (or pickled sugar-free fish)	0	0	0
1 cup shredded iceberg lettuce	1	1	0
1 1/2 teaspoons capers	0	0	0
1 cup bean sprouts	6	2	4
Vinegar and oil dressing (1 teaspoon vinegar and			
1 teaspoon olive oil)	0	0	0
2 ounces Swiss cheese slices	2	0	2
Breakfast TOTAL*	**9**	**3**	**6**
LUNCH			
Large spinach salad with:			
3 cups fresh spinach	3	2	1
1 ounce mixed unsalted nuts	7	3	4
3 tablespoons dry-roasted sunflower seeds	6	3	3
2 tablespoons onions, sliced thin	2	0	2
vinegar and oil dressing (1 tablespoon vinegar and			
1 tablespoon olive oil)	1	0	1
1 ounce blue cheese	1	0	1
1 tablespoon crumbled bacon (or bacon bits)	0	0	0
Lunch TOTAL*	**19**	**8**	**11**
DINNER			
6 ounces grilled burgers (or sausages or vegetarian burgers)			
topped with:	0	0	0
2 tablespoons onions (not chopped), grilled	2	0	2
1/2 cup mushrooms, grilled	2	0	2
1 cup sautéed zucchini	3	1	2
2 cups mixed salad greens with:	3	1	2
vinegar and oil dressing (2 teaspoons vinegar and			
2 teaspoons olive oil)	0	0	0
1 cup sugar-free gelatin dessert with:	2	0	2
1 tablespoon whipped cream	0	0	0
Dinner TOTAL*	**12**	**3**	**9**
SNACKS			
2 ounces cheddar cheese (or other hard cheese)	1	0	1
TOTAL FOR DAY*	**41**	**14**	**27**

▦ DAY 4 ▦

(Pharmafoods in boldface)

	CARBS, GRAMS	FIBER, GRAMS	NET CARBS	% MONO
BREAKFAST				
2 ounces string cheese	2	0	2	25
1 ounce mixed unsalted **nuts**	7	3	4	61
1 hard-boiled egg	1	0	1	38
Breakfast TOTAL*	**9**	**3**	**6**	**43**
LUNCH				
4 slices extra-lean deli ham wrapped in lettuce leaves	1	0	1	47
Homemade coleslaw with:				
2 cups chopped **cabbage**	10	4	6	—
1 tablespoon mayonnaise	0	0	0	27
1 large sour pickle	3	2	1	—
Lunch TOTAL*	**14**	**6**	**8**	**35**
DINNER				
Homemade meatloaf made with:				
6 ounces ground beef	0	0	0	44
¼ cup wheat bran	9	6	3	—
1 cup **zucchini**	3	1	2	—
½ cup **broccoli**	4	2	2	—
1 tablespoon butter for vegetables	0	0	0	29
Berries and *fruit salad dressing* made with:				
¼ cup plain **yogurt**	2	0	2	25
½ cup fresh **strawberries**	5	2	3	—
1 packet sweetener	1	0	1	—
Dinner TOTAL*	**25**	**12**	**13**	**37**
SNACKS				
2 ounces cheddar cheese (or other hard cheese)	1	0	1	29
TOTAL FOR DAY*	**49**	**20**	**29**	**36**

Phase 1: Getting Started

▨ DAY 5 ▨
(Pharmafoods in boldface)

	CARBS, GRAMS	FIBER, GRAMS	NET CARBS	% MONO
BREAKFAST				
1 cup plain *yogurt* (sweetened if desired) with:	4	0	4	25
2 tablespoons **sunflower seeds**	4	2	2	20
1 ounce mixed unsalted **nuts**	7	3	4	61
Breakfast TOTAL*	**15**	**4**	**11**	**42**
LUNCH				
Coleslaw made with:				
1¹/₂ cups **cabbage**	7	3	4	—
1 tablespoon mayonnaise	0	0	0	27
Cucumber salad made with:				
1 cup cucumber	3	1	2	—
vinegar and oil dressing				
(2 teaspoons vinegar and 2 teaspoons olive oil)	0	0	0	74
1 piece of high-fiber crispbread** with	6	1	5**	—
1 tablespoon natural **peanut butter**	3	1	2	50
Lunch TOTAL*	**20**	**6**	**14**	**48**
DINNER				
6 ounces grilled salmon	0	0	0	48
¹/₂ cup green beans with:	5	2	3	—
1 ounce slivered **almonds**	3	2	1	63
¹/₂ cup **zucchini** (sprinkle with some of almonds if desired)	2	1	1	
2 cups mixed salad greens with:	3	1	2	—
lemon and oil dressing (2 teaspoons lemon juice and				
2 teaspoons olive oil)	1	0	1	74
Fruit salad made with:				
¹/₄ cup **cantaloupe**	4	0	4	—
¹/₄ of a **kiwi**	3	1	2	—
Dinner TOTAL*	**20**	**6**	**14**	**56**
SNACKS				
2 ounces cheddar cheese (or other hard cheese)	1	0	1	29
TOTAL FOR THE DAY*	**56**	**17**	**39**	**45**

■ DAY 6 ■

(Pharmafoods in boldface)

	CARBS, GRAMS	FIBER, GRAMS	NET CARBS	% MONO
BREAKFAST				
Chocolate kefir shake made with:				
1 cup **kefir**	4	0	4	29
1½ teaspoons **flaxseed**, freshly ground	2	2	0	20
½ ounce unsalted **nuts**	4	1	1	61
1 tablespoon unsweetened cocoa powder	3	2	1	25
2 packets sugar substitute (or to taste)	2	0	2	–
Breakfast TOTAL*	**14**	**5**	**9**	**39**
LUNCH				
Vegetarian salad with:				
3 cups mixed salad greens	5	2	3	–
1 cup **broccoli**	8	5	3	–
4 ounces **tofu**	2	2	0	22
½ **avocado**	7	5	2	63
1 tablespoon **sunflower seeds**	2	2	0	20
Vinegar and oil dressing (1 tablespoon vinegar and				
1 tablespoon olive oil)	1	0	1	–
Deviled eggs made with:				
2 eggs	1	0	1	48
1 tablespoon mayonnaise	0	0	0	27
Lunch TOTAL*	**26**	**14**	**12**	**48**
DINNER				
Stir-fry made with:				
5 ounces shrimp (or meat or fish or tofu)	1	0	1	20
1 cup mushrooms	3	1	2	–
1 cup **broccoli**	8	5	3	–
1 tablespoon chopped **onions**	1	0	1	–
2 slices fresh ginger	1	0	1	–
1 tablespoon olive oil for frying	0	0	0	74
Served on:				
1 cup riced **cauliflower**	5	3	2	–
Rhubarb and berry compote made with:				
¼ cup diced rhubarb stalks	1	1	0	–
¼ cup fresh **strawberries**	3	1	2	–
1 tablespoon whipped cream	0	0	0	29

	CARBS, GRAMS	FIBER, GRAMS	NET CARBS	% MONO
2 packets sweetener (or to taste)	2	0	2	—
Dinner TOTAL*	**25**	**10**	**15**	**55**
SNACKS				
2 ounces cheddar cheese (or other hard cheese)	1	0	1	29
TOTAL FOR THE DAY*	**67**	**29**	**38**	**45**

▓ DAY 7 ▓
(Pharmafoods in boldface)

	CARBS, GRAMS	FIBER, GRAMS	NET CARBS	% MONO
BREAKFAST				
2 crispbreads** (or low-carb toast)	12	3	9**	—
2 tablespoons natural **peanut butter** (or farmers cheese)	6	2	4	50
Breakfast TOTAL*	**18**	**5**	**13**	**50**
LUNCH				
8 ounces plain **yogurt** with:	4	0	4	25
1 ounce mixed **nuts**	7	3	4	61
Steamed vegetable plate made with:				
¹/₂ cup **broccoli**	4	2	2	—
¹/₂ cup **cauliflower**	2	2	0	—
¹/₂ cup **Brussels sprouts**	4	2	2	—
1 tablespoon **flaxseed**, freshly ground	4	3	1	20
1 tablespoon olive oil	0	0	0	74
Lunch TOTAL*	**26**	**12**	**14**	**52**
DINNER				
Grilled chicken breast	0	0	0	39
1 cup (fresh) **spinach** or ¹/₂ cup (cooked)	1	1	0	—
Salad made with:				
2 cups mixed salad greens	3	1	2	—
2 chopped **scallions**	4	1	3	—
¹/₂ **avocado**	7	5	2	63
Vinegar and oil dressing (2 teaspoons vinegar and				
2 teaspoons olive oil)	0	0	0	74
Chocolate almond ricotta dessert with:				
¹/₂ cup ricotta cheese	4	0	4	28
¹/₂ ounce chopped **almonds**	3	2	1	63
1¹/₂ teaspoons cocoa powder	1	1	0	25
1 packet sweetener (or to taste)	1	0	1	—

Few drops of almond or banana flavoring	0	0	0	—
Dinner TOTAL*	**24**	**11**	**13**	**50**
SNACKS				
1 ounce cheddar cheese (or other hard cheese)	0	0	0	29
1/2 ounce almonds	3	2	1	63
Snack TOTAL*	**3**	**2**	**1**	**41**
TOTAL FOR THE DAY*	**72**	**28**	**44**	**50**

◆ As noted in the text, you don't need to follow these menus to succeed on this diet. They are provided simply as a guide to show you the types of foods you might want to eat during the first three days and as you transition from a diet that is simply low in carbohydrate to a diet that is healthy and contains sufficient fiber and vitamins and minerals. They also suggest how you can keep track of the carbohydrates and fat in your food.

You can also use the food suggested here but alter the amounts to satisfy your own individual appetite. The menus range from about 1,500 to about 2,000 calories, but you may need more or less than those amounts. If you're satisfied with less, stop eating and give your dog a treat. If you're still hungry, eat more of the noncarby foods or have more of the recommended snacks until you're full, but not stuffed.

If you're eating less, eat less of the carby foods or those low in monosaturated fat (e.g., eggs, commercial mayonnaise, butter, cocoa powder, or cream; flaxseed is low in monounsaturated fat but contains beneficial omega-3 fatty acids and should not be avoided). If you're eating more, choose the foods that don't contain carbohydrates and are high in monounsaturated fat (e.g., olives, olive oil, avocados, nuts, homemade mayonnaise). Use the Net Carbs and % Mono columns to help you decide which foods to eat more or less of.

After the first week, you should be able to plan your own menus following the rules of the diet. If at first you find it difficult to keep track of everything, it would be a good idea to take a daily calcium supplement as well as a standard multivitamin pill to make sure you're getting the vitamins and minerals you need. Later, as you've adapted to more vegetables and dairy products (yogurt, kefir, and cheese), this shouldn't be necessary.

◆ For the first three days, the focus is on net carbohydrate content, and you may be eating more saturated fat than you would like. Don't worry about it. It's only for a few days.

After the first three days, you begin to focus on nutritious monounsaturated fat, fiber, and pharmafoods. The fiber and mono fat amounts or percentages are shown for each ingredient, meal, and day's total. The pharmafoods are emphasized with boldface. If you want to have more of the pharmafoods or foods that are high in these nutrients, go ahead, as long as you don't exceed the carb counts.

◆ Men should add a little tomato to each day's menu because of the beneficial lycopenes in tomatos that help to prevent prostate cancer.

◆ The analysis of the dairy foods is for full-fat products. You can decrease your intake of saturated fat by using reduced-fat products, but you'll reduce your intake of monounsaturated fat as well. Remember, avoid fat-free products, which are often filled with carbohydrate fillers. You can increase your monounsaturated fat intake by using mayonnaise made with olive oil or canola oil instead of the standard commercial mayonnaise used in these analyses, by eating more avocado, or by using more olive oil on salads and vegetables.

◆ These menus should give you an idea of one way to keep track of your carbohydrate and monounsaturated fat intake. But you don't need to get this complicated. Use whatever system works for you.

◆ We have suggested using cheese for snacks because this will ensure that you get at least 1,000 milligrams of calcium a day using these menus. If you'd like to substitute another high-calcium snack like fortified low-carb soy milk or yogurt instead of the cheese, that's fine. Or if you'd rather use lower-calcium snacks and take a calcium supplement, you can do that, too. If your hunger is satisfied without the cheese snacks, it would be a good idea to add a calcium supplement as well.

If you do choose the cheese, you don't need to use cheddar. Most hard cheeses contain about the same amount of calcium, so vary your cheeses if you like. And of course you don't need to eat all two ounces at once. You can eat some when you get hungry between meals, or you can grate it over vegetables with a meal. If you've eaten all the cheese and you're still hungry between meals, see the list of snack suggestions in this chapter. Remember, you can eat all you like as long as you don't exceed the carbohydrate limit.

◆ Items in italic have recipes in the Recipe section.

◆ Dashes mean the amount of fat is insignificant.

◆ One ounce of nuts is about two rounded tablespoons, or about twenty-two almonds.

* Note that because of rounding off, the totals for the meal and for the day may be slightly different from what you get when you add yourself. This is because the computer is using more decimal places than are shown in the report. For example, 1.6 + 1.6 + 1.6 = 4.6, which rounds to 5. But the data would be shown as 2 + 2 + 2 = 5.

** Carb counts on crispbreads vary a lot. Get the brand with the lowest count you can find.

If you'd rather plan your own menus, that's fine. If you want to eat the sample breakfast for Day 1 for all three days of Phase 1, that's fine. If you want to substitute one of the dinner menus for lunch, that's fine. Do what works for you. However, try not to go from almost no fiber to 30 grams too suddenly or you may have a gastrointestinal rebellion. The menus are designed to help you gradually transition to a higher fiber consumption.

Table 4.5 shows the nutritional analysis of the Day 7 menu, showing that it has satisfied the requirements of the Four Corners Diet: less than 50 grams of net carbohydrates per day, less than 15 grams of net carbohydrates per meal, 50 percent monounsaturated fat, less than 40 grams of saturated fat, and more than 15 grams of fiber. Note that if you don't add salt to your food, the sodium content is also well below the recommended limit for those needing to limit salt intake. Calcium is slightly higher than the recommended 1000 milligrams, and levels of other nutrients are at reasonable levels. This diet is healthy!

TABLE 4.5
Nutritional Analysis of Day 7*

NUTRIENT	QUANTITY
Calories	2,022
Carbohydrate	72 grams
Dietary fiber	28 grams
Net carbs	44 grams
Sugars	[25] grams
Starch	[18] grams
Soluble fiber	[5] grams
Net carbs (breakfast)	13 grams
Net carbs (lunch)	14 grams
Net carbs (snacks)	1 grams
Net carbs (dinner)	13 grams
Fat	139 grams
Saturated fat	38 grams
Monounsaturated fat	69 grams (50% of fat)
Polyunsaturated fat	23 grams
Cholesterol	307 milligrams
Protein	127 grams
Calcium	1083 milligrams
Magnesium	467 milligrams
Sodium	895 milligrams
Potassium	3424 milligrams
Iron	12.2 milligrams
Phosphorus	1695 milligrams
Vitamin A_IU	[2603] IU
Vitamin C	170.9 milligrams
Vitamin E	[21] milligrams
Vitamin D	[3] IU
TAG	[119] grams

* See notes at end of Appendix II for an explanation of the brackets and TAG.

Table 4.6 is a shopping list to help you get started if you decide to follow these menus.

TABLE 4.6
Shopping List Week 1
❖

The amounts in parentheses show the minimal amount you'd need if you were going to follow the amounts shown in the menus exactly, for one person. If you think you have a larger appetite, get more of the noncarby foods.

FOOD	AMOUNT TO PURCHASE
Avocado	1 avocado
Bacon bits, real bacon	1 jar (1 tablespoon, or make crumbled bacon bits yourself)
Bacon	$\frac{1}{2}$ pound (3 slices)
Bean sprouts	$\frac{1}{2}$ pound (1 cup)
Beans, green	1 pound ($1\frac{1}{2}$ cups)
Beef, ground	1 pound (12 ounces)
Broccoli	2 pounds (4 cups)
Brussels sprouts	$\frac{1}{4}$ pound ($\frac{1}{4}$ cup)
Butter	$\frac{1}{2}$ pound ($4\frac{1}{2}$ teaspoons)
Cabbage	1 head ($3\frac{1}{2}$ cups)
Cantaloupe	1 fruit or 1 slice ($\frac{1}{4}$ cup)
Capers	1 bottle ($\frac{1}{2}$ tablespoon)
Cauliflower	1 pound ($2\frac{1}{2}$ cups)
Cheese, blue	1 package (1 ounce)
Cheese, cheddar	1 pound (15 ounces)
Cheese, ricotta	$\frac{1}{2}$ pint ($\frac{1}{2}$ cup)
Cheese, string	1 package (2 ounces)
Cheese, Swiss	1 package (3 ounces)
Chicken breast with skin	2 large chicken breasts
Chocolate-flavored soda, sugar-free	1 can
Cocoa powder, unsweetened	1 can ($1\frac{1}{2}$ tablespoons)
Crispbread, high-fiber	1 package (3 pieces)
Cream, whipping	$\frac{1}{2}$ pint ($3\frac{1}{2}$ tablespoons)
Cucumber	2 medium or 1 large (2 cups)
Cucumber pickles, sour	1 jar (2 pickles)
Eggs	1 dozen (9 eggs)
Flaxseed	1 package ($1\frac{1}{2}$ tablespoons)
Flavoring, banana or almond	1 bottle (few drops)
Gelatin dessert, sugar-free	1 or 2 packages (2 cups)
Ginger root, raw	1 piece (2 slices)

FOOD	AMOUNT TO PURCHASE
Ham, sliced deli	1 packet (4 slices; about 4 ounces)
Kefir	8 ounces (1 cup)
Kiwi	1 fruit ($\frac{1}{4}$ kiwi)
Lemons	1 lemon (2 teaspoons of juice)
Lettuce, iceberg	1 head (3 cups)
Mayonnaise	1 jar (3 tablespoons)
Mushrooms, fresh	1 pound ($1\frac{1}{2}$ cups)
Nuts, slivered almonds	1 package (2 ounces)
Nuts, mixed	1 package ($4\frac{1}{2}$ ounces)
Oil, olive	1 bottle (about 8 tablespoons, but you want to have a lot on hand)
Olives, ripe	1 can (10 olives)
Onions	1 pound (5 tablespoons)
Peanut butter, natural	1 jar (3 tablespoons)
Pork, ham	1 piece cooked (2 ounces)
Pork roast	1 roast (6 ounces)
Rhubarb	1 piece or bunch ($\frac{1}{4}$ cup)
Salad dressing, ranch	1 bottle (1 tablespoon) (check ingredients for carbs)
Salad greens mix	Enough to make 13 cups for the whole week. Buy daily if possible and vary the greens.
Salmon fillet	$\frac{1}{2}$ pound (6 ounces)
Salmon, smoked	1 package (4 ounces)
Sauerkraut	1 package or can ($\frac{1}{2}$ cup)
Scallions	2 scallions (wash carefully)
Shrimp	6 ounces
Sour cream	1 carton (2 tablespoons)
Spinach, fresh	$\frac{1}{2}$ pound (4 cups)
Strawberries	1 container ($\frac{3}{4}$ cup)
Sugar substitute	1 box of packets (at least 6 packets)
Sunflower seeds, unsalted	1 package (6 tablespoons)
Tofu	$\frac{1}{2}$ pound (4 ounces)
Tuna, canned, in oil	1 can (6 ounces)
Turkey breast, cooked	$\frac{1}{4}$ pound (2 ounces)
Vinegar	1 bottle (about 4 tablespoons)
Wheat bran	1 package ($\frac{1}{4}$ cup)
Yogurt, plain	3 containers ($2\frac{1}{2}$ cups)
Zucchini	2 medium ($2\frac{1}{2}$ cups)

If you're able to calculate carb counts yourself and you'd like to do mix-and-match meals on your own, here are some more suggestions:

Breakfast Suggestions
 ❖ Plain kefir drink—with nuts and sunflower kernels on the side
 ❖ Plain yogurt mixed with nuts, cinnamon, no-calorie sweetener to taste
 ❖ Nuts and cheese cubes or string cheese
 ❖ Breakfast parfait with layers of plain yogurt, very high-fiber cereal (BranBuds, All-Bran), sunflower seeds

Lunch Suggestions
 ❖ Cheeseburgers without the bun, side salad, no-carbohydrate condiments
 ❖ Stir-fried vegetables in oil and chicken breast
 ❖ Cheese-stuffed portobello mushrooms and salad
 ❖ Assorted cold cuts and cucumber salad with sour cream
 ❖ Hot dogs or bratwurst without the bun, sauerkraut, and dill pickle

Dinner Suggestions
 ❖ Grilled lean steak, large spinach salad, stir-fried zucchini
 ❖ Baked whitefish, asparagus, stir-fried mushrooms, mixed greens salad
 ❖ Stir-fried lean beef and Chinese vegetables (no rice)
 ❖ Dinner-sized Cobb salad with cubed smoked turkey, ham, cheese, chopped egg on mixed greens

Desserts and Snacks
 ❖ Flavored coffees (no syrups), no-calorie sweeteners, and cream
 ❖ Flavored sodas—club soda or seltzer water mixed with sugar-free flavored syrups
 ❖ Cheese cubes and nuts (limit nuts to ½ cup per day)
 ❖ Ricotta cheese and cinnamon, or other flavoring, no-calorie sweetener
 ❖ Hard-boiled eggs
 ❖ Chicken drumsticks and wings
 ❖ Kefir or yogurt shake; use no-calorie sweeteners
 ❖ Guacamole on celery, radishes, cucumbers, broccoli, or pork rinds
 ❖ Olives
 ❖ Sugar-free gelatin desserts
 ❖ Vegetable, beef, and chicken broths

Just remember the essentials: No more than 15 grams of net carbohydrates per meal. No more than 50 grams of net carbohydrates per day. Eat enough other food so you're not hungry. Don't skip meals. Don't eat any food that isn't listed in Table 4.3.

Be sure to have canned tuna, cheese cubes, hard-boiled eggs, and chicken wings around in case you get "shaky." This can happen if your blood sugar level drops too low. If you're overweight and your diet has been high in carbohydrates, it's possible that you have high circulating insulin levels. When you suddenly stop eating carbohydrates, it will take a day or so for your body to stop producing high levels of insulin. In the meantime, you might have a drop in blood sugar that you'll feel as shakiness or weakness. You should eat something if you feel that way. High-protein snacks are best. This problem should abate as your body becomes accustomed to the new way of eating.

It may be very difficult at first to give up your carby friends, and you may wonder why you have to go through this very strict first-phase transition diet. Theoretically, you don't. But if you don't, it may take a longer time for your body to change into a fat-burning machine and you may give in to temptation and lose your motivation for the diet.

The purpose of the transition diet is to deprive the body of almost all carbohydrates and force it to switch over to burning fat for fuel as quickly as possible. This requires totally different enzyme machinery than the carbohydrate factories. Once your body is convinced that the carbohydrates are not coming back, it will put all its efforts into creating enough capacity to satisfy all your energy needs from fats. That means not only the very efficient handling of dietary fats, but also the ability to mobilize that fat reserve it's been carefully sculpting on your thighs, waist, and hips for the past few years. It's as though your body has been saving for a rainy day and it has just started to pour.

Once all this machinery is in place, you will have turned your body into a fat-burning furnace. Need some energy? Take it from my butt. Need more energy? Take it from my thighs. Your enzyme machinery can handle large quantities of dietary fat, and it will have the ability to mobilize your entire fat stores. You will no longer have to put the feedbag on to get energy. You have it on demand, gushing forth from your fat cells like a newly found oil well.

So, these first three days may be hard, but remember, it gets easier as time goes on. And you'll be happy with the results.

▶ IF YOU HAVE DIABETES

IF YOU HAVE Diabetes, it is especially important to consult your doctor before embarking on a drastic change of diet, especially if you are taking insulin or one of the sulfonylurea drugs that can make your blood sugar levels go too low.

The dosages of these drugs were undoubtedly calculated on the assumption that you would be eating a very high-carbohydrate American Diabetes Association diet. If you take enough insulin to cover 60 grams of carbohydrates in a meal and you eat only 15, your blood sugar will go too low, even to a dangerous level. The same can be true with a sulfonylurea drug.

Other drugs, such as metformin, do not reduce your blood sugar directly, but they reduce your insulin resistance, and you may have to cut back on these drugs as well.

One problem you may have is a physician or certified diabetes educator (CDE) who does not approve of low-carbohydrate diets and refuses to give you any help in this area. If this happens to you, try to find a doctor or CDE with a more open mind.

If you have no choice in health care people, you'll have to do this yourself. If you're taking insulin, you're probably already accustomed to adjusting your insulin dosages slightly, depending on what you eat. But the changes you're about to undertake are more drastic than changing from two slices of bread to one.

Be careful. Be alert for signs of low blood sugar (which can include shakiness, sweating, rapid heartbeat, hunger, irritability, confusion, anxiety, and a feeling of nervousness or impending doom). Use your meter to measure your blood glucose levels more often than usual to make sure the diet isn't making you go too low. If it is, reduce your insulin dosages or take less of your sulfonylurea drug.

Remember, *low blood sugar can be lethal.* Slightly elevated blood sugar levels for a short period of time won't be harmful. So err on the side of caution. Let your blood sugar levels get too high rather than too low. Work with a doctor or a CDE if you can.

FIVE

Phase 2:
Making the Diet Healthy

CONGRATULATIONS! YOU'VE PASSED the first test. You've gotten through three days of eating very little carbohydrate, and now your body is beginning to burn fat for energy.

Now it's time to focus on making your diet healthy by adding the other three corners of the diet: monounsaturated fat, fiber, and pharmafoods.

CORNER 2:
MONOUNSATURATED FAT

SATURATED FAT HAS been associated with hypertension, diabetes, and heart disease. *Association* is not the same as *cause*, and some of these associations are controversial; there are no studies showing such associations in people who are also limiting their carbohydrate intake. Nevertheless, in this diet we are taking a conservative approach. We emphasize monounsaturated fat, which has not been found to have the associations we mentioned.

You can have some saturated fat in your diet, up to about 40 grams a day, depending on your size and energy needs. If you're not eating much carbohydrate, you're going to be eating more fat, so it's important to make sure it's the right kind.

Your goal should be to make 50 percent of your fatty acids the right kind, the monounsaturated fatty acids, which from now on we will call MUFAs. This may sound complicated, but it's not as hard as it seems. Table 4.2 in Chapter 4 lists MUFA percentages of some common foods, as well as their carbohydrate content. Note that most meats, fish, and chicken already contain more than 40 percent MUFAs. Hence, supplementing your diet with a few foods containing very high levels of MUFAs can easily bring you over the 50 percent level.

On the other hand, dairy products have less than 30 percent MUFAs. So if you eat a lot of cheese, you will have to eat a lot more of the high-MUFA foods. (You might think you could easily reduce your saturated fat intake by eating low-fat cheeses. They do have less saturated fat, but they also have less monounsaturated fat, and the ratio is about the same. *Avoid the fat-free cheeses*, which are usually bulked up with sugars and other carbohydrates.)

What are the high-MUFA foods? These include olive oil, canola oil, avocado, and most nuts. Yes, that's right, *nuts*. You may have given up eating nuts, thinking that they are a fattening food because of their high fat content. Not so! Nuts are an excellent source of the right fats— MUFAs—and fiber.

Now you can rediscover the taste and crunch of nuts and seeds. You can use ground-up nuts to make pie crusts. You can add chopped nuts to yogurt. You can sprinkle your vegetables with chopped nuts. You can add nuts to a high-fiber cereal. You can use nuts for snacks. There are myriad ways to use these nutritious little gems.

Avocados are also high in MUFAs. Guacamole and other avocado salads are a great-tasting way to increase your MUFA intake. Try a chicken taco salad with extra guacamole. You can even use avocados to make a dessert (see Recipe section).

Don't panic about the 50 percent goal. Remember it's just a goal, and you may not reach the goal every day. Just do your best. Make sure you have olive oil, canola oil, nuts and seeds, olives, and avocados readily available in your kitchen.

Trim meats of excess fat, and skim soups and stews of any fats you can see on the top. If you prepare them ahead of time, the fat will solidify in the refrigerator and be much easier to remove. Emphasize fish and grilled lean meats and chicken. Eat less of fatty meats, sausages, and high-saturated-fat cold cuts like bologna.

Get into the habit of dressing salads with olive oil, stir-frying vegetables and meat with oil, dressing your vegetables with oil instead of butter, eating avocados, and snacking on nuts and seeds.

Here are a few tips on how to increase the percentage of MUFAs in your diet:

❖ A meal of steak and a salad with olive oil and vinegar dressing will have over 50 percent MUFAs.

❖ You can increase MUFAs in a kefir shake by adding 1 tablespoon of canola oil.

❖ A meal of a two-egg omelet with cheddar cheese is acceptable provided you fry it in olive oil.

❖ Snacking on nuts and seeds and eating less meat helps your daily totals.

CORNER 3:
FIBER

YOUR DIET NEEDS a lot of fiber, both the soluble and the insoluble kind. Many people get their fiber from beans and whole grains, but beans (except for soybeans) and whole grains contain too many carbohydrates for you. So how are you supposed to get enough fiber to reach your goal of 25 grams?

Vegetables contain fiber, and many vegetables are also low in carbohydrates. Some high-fiber vegetables include avocados, bamboo shoots, broccoli, Brussels sprouts, cauliflower, cabbage, green beans, and spinach.

Vegetables that are especially high in soluble fiber include okra, eggplant, and nopal cactus.

Other good sources of fiber are nuts and seeds. However, you will probably find that you'll need to add some very high-fiber foods such as bran to your diet to reach your goal.

Any kind of bran can be used. Corn bran has the least carbohydrate and is the tastiest of the brans, but is difficult to buy in retail amounts. Wheat bran is readily available and is fairly cheap. Rice bran has a little more carbohydrate than wheat bran but is a lifesaver for those with a wheat allergy. Oat bran has more soluble fiber than wheat bran and has a tastier flavor, but it also has more carbohydrates.

Some supermarkets stock brans in the section with flour and other dry bulk items. You may have to find a health food store in order to purchase bran.

Don't confuse products whose labels say they contain "whole wheat" or "wheat germ" with products containing wheat bran. They're not the same. There is little or no fiber in such products, and they can't substitute for real bran. Likewise, don't think that "natural oats" or most "bran cereals" contain any meaningful fiber. Check the label for fiber content before you buy and make sure you're buying the right thing.

You can use bran to make pancakes, muffins, waffles, cereals, and breads (see Recipe section). Use wheat bran as an extender in meatloaf and meatballs and other recipes that call for bread crumbs.

Use your imagination. Just keep track of the carbohydrates as you do, and make sure the *net* carbohydrates in your final products fit into your meal allowance.

Ground flaxseeds are also a wonderful source of both soluble and insoluble fiber. They are also loaded with phytoestrogens as well as beneficial omega-6 and omega-3 unsaturated fatty acids. Many modern diets are deficient in omega-3 fatty acids, which are found in high amounts in seafoods. Flaxseed has one of the highest levels of omega-3 fatty acids among plant foods, as well as antioxidants and substances that may offer protection against some kinds of cancer.

The omega-3 fatty acids oxidize readily when they're exposed to air; we say the product is *rancid*. The hull of the flaxseed protects it from air. Hence it's better to grind your flaxseeds in a coffee grinder right before you use them. If you don't have a grinder (you can buy one for about $10), keep the bag of flax meal tightly closed in your refrigerator.

You can use flaxseed to make a quick hot cereal (see Recipe section). The flaxseed does have a slightly bitter aftertaste, so you might want to add some cinnamon to the cereal. Adding flax to oat bran increases the nutrient content while preserving the taste of the oats.

Psyllium husks are considered a natural laxative because of their fiber content. You can also use psyllium powder—or guar or xanthan gums, other soluble fibers—as thickening agents in gravies and stews. Psyllium is also an excellent binder for meatloaf or meatballs. You can also add it to yogurt to give it a creamier taste.

If you need to hide psyllium powder in order to get it down, try sugar-free flavored psyllium products stirred into club soda. Or stir it into a low-carb breakfast shake.

Check the fiber contents of foods to maximize the amount of fiber you take in every day. Some premade cereals that are extra high in fiber are suitable for the Four Corners Diet. One such commercial cereal has 14 grams of fiber per half cup.

If you combine a half cup of this cereal with half an ounce of sunflower seeds, half an ounce of walnuts, a little no-calorie sweetener, and some whole cream or kefir, you will have an excellent breakfast with more than 15 grams of fiber and less than 15 grams of net carbohydrates.

Remember that your goal is at least 25 grams of fiber a day. But a high-fiber diet can also result in some gas, and you shouldn't attempt to reach the 25-gram goal right away. Go slowly. Add a little more fiber to your diet every day until you get close to your goal. This will give the colon bacteria that produce the gas enough time to adapt to your new way of eating so the intestinal disturbances will be minor.

Table 5.1 lists some foods with a lot of fiber and a relatively low net-carbohydrate content.

TABLE 5.1
High-Fiber, Low-Carbohydrate Foods*
❖

Most of the carbohydrate in these foods is 50 percent or more fiber.

FOOD	GRAMS OF CARBS PER 100 GRAMS	GRAMS OF FIBER PER 100 GRAMS	NET CARBS PER 100 GRAMS	PERCENTAGE FIBER
Corn bran (available only in carload lots)	86	86	0	100
Wheat bran**	67	47	20	70
Rice bran**	50	21	29	42
Psyllium husks	81	72	9	89
Flaxseed	34	28	6	82
Gums such as guar and xanthan	Not in USDA database	Almost 100% fiber	—	—
Extra-high-fiber breakfast cereals†	Check labels	Check labels	—	—
Extra-high-fiber crispbreads†	Check labels	Check labels	—	—
Raspberries	12	7	5	58
Avocado	7	5	2	71
Okra	6	3	3	50
Broccoli	5	3	2	60
Bamboo shoots	3	3	0	100
Brussels sprouts	8	4	4	50
Cauliflower	4	3	1	75
Cabbage	4	2	2	50
Green beans	8	3	5	38
Spinach	4	3	1	75
Collards	6	3	3	50
Nopal cactus	3	2	1	67
Eggplant	6	3	3	50
Almonds	20	12	8	60
Four Corners recipes made with added bran	—	—	—	—

* Note that these values are based on 100 grams. This means that dry ingredients such as the brans have a lot of carbs per 100 grams. Serving sizes would be much smaller. A half cup of wheat bran has about 33 grams. Also remember that small numbers are only estimates because rounding off can have a relatively large effect.

** The composition of brans differs a lot from manufacturer to manufacturer. Oat bran contains about 66 grams of carbs and only 15 grams of fiber per 100 grams and hence is not as beneficial as the other brans. Wheat bran is better than rice bran unless you're allergic to wheat.

† Check labels. Some have a lot more net carbs than others.

CORNER 4:
PHARMAFOODS

Probiotic Foods

You are probably already familiar with the probiotics yogurt and buttermilk. Sauerkraut and other fermented vegetables are also probiotics. If you are from eastern Europe or the Middle East, you are familiar with kefir as well. You might refer to it as "drinkable" yogurt. Kefir originated in eastern Europe centuries ago. It is a milk product made from kefir "grains." These grains consist of a mass of bacteria and yeast, polysaccharides, and curds of milk protein that is then incubated with milk. The end composition generally has from two to seven active microbial types.

You should try to have at least 1 cup of yogurt, kefir, or buttermilk every day. Of the three live-culture products, kefir may be the healthiest, because in addition to the beneficial *lactobacilli* found in the other two, kefir also contains "friendly" yeasts, which help to prevent overgrowth of other, less friendly forms of yeast.

Kefir has been widely used in western Europe, and today commercial kefir is available in many American health food stores. It may even be found in your local supermarket. If not, it's easy to make (see Recipe section). If you are trying to follow a vegan version of this diet, you can make your products from soy milk.

The bacteria that convert milk to yogurt do so by converting the milk sugar, lactose, into lactic acid. It's this lactic acid that curdles the milk and makes the yogurt both solid and tart. In one brand of kefir made by a national manufacturer, only 1 percent of the lactose from the milk remains in the kefir product.

This means two things. First, even if you're lactose intolerant, you should be able to tolerate these probiotic foods. Daily consumption of yogurt colonizes the intestine with these friendly bacteria, which should help you handle the small amounts of lactose remaining in the product.

Second, because the lactic acid doesn't raise your blood sugar levels as other sugars do, you don't need to count all the carbohydrates on the food labels of these probiotic foods.

Why is this? It's because the carbohydrate in foods is often measured by what is called the *difference* method. This means they measure the protein, fat, ash, and water and assume that everything else — the difference — is carbohydrates. This system works well for many foods but not for those containing a lot of something like lactic acid. We don't count the lactic acid as a carbohydrate.

You can subtract 1 gram of carbohydrate for each ounce of these probiotic foods you eat. Thus, for a standard 8-ounce container of plain yogurt, which usually says it has about 12 grams of carbohydrates, you need to count only 4. This is not just speculation. Dr. Goldberg has actually measured the carbohydrate content of yogurt in his own laboratory.

When you go to buy commercial yogurt and kefir, look for plain, unsweetened, or artificially sweetened varieties. Many Americans are accustomed to eating yogurt only when it's mixed with very sweet fruits or jams. But peoples who have eaten such products for generations usually eat them unsweetened.

In fact, when you tell your grandmother about your new diet, she may tell you it's not new at all. Maybe she'll share with you yogurt- or kefir-making stories from her childhood.

Also, make sure the plain yogurt you buy contains live cultures. We prefer yogurt and kefir that is made from growth hormone–free organic milk.

Unsweetened yogurt makes an excellent salad with cucumbers (see Recipe section) and can also be added to soups, vegetable dishes, dips, and toppings in place of sour cream. Just be careful to add it to hot dishes after cooking so it doesn't separate. There are also many, many ways you can eat yogurt as a dessert, using artificial sweeteners and a few berries, nuts, and all kinds of flavorings. In fact, when you buy plain yogurt and make your own flavors, you're going to have a much more varied and interesting variety than the few fruit flavors you'll find available at the supermarket.

You can make your own yogurt with either regular or reduced-fat or even skim milk, depending on how low you want your consumption of saturated fat to be. Made with whole milk, the product is smoother, but you can add some psyllium, guar, or xanthan gum to the lower-fat varieties to give a smoother taste. As always, when buying commercial plain yogurt, make sure to read the labels. Some commercial skim-milk yogurts are thickened with additional lactose-containing milk solids and cornstarch, both of which add to the carbohydrate content. Making skim-milk yogurt at home eliminates that problem.

You can also make cheese from kefir and yogurt (see Recipe section). You may even be able to buy such cheeses ready-made.

Finally, remember that milk products are a good source of calcium.

Yogurt and kefir made from milk that has been supplemented with calcium and vitamin D have additional health benefits.

Other Pharmafoods

In order to be as healthy as possible, you want to get as many vitamins and minerals from your food as possible. Sure, you can supplement with vitamin pills. But vitamin pills contain only the nutrients that someone has determined are essential for life. There may be nutrients in fresh foods that are very beneficial but haven't yet been isolated and offered in pills.

Thus you should eat *at least* five servings of assorted vegetables every day, preferably from the *other pharmafoods* group. If you want, you can substitute one serving (½ cup) of a high-fiber fruit with a low net-carbohydrate count (berries, for example).

These vegetables should include a variety of dark green, leafy, and yellow vegetables to provide natural sources of many vitamins and minerals. Whenever possible, use unprocessed forms of foods, which are more likely to contain beneficial vitamins and other health-promoting nutrients. Men should try to eat a little bit of tomato every day, either fresh or cooked in marinara sauce or in salsa, because of the anti–prostate cancer properties of the lycopenes in tomatoes.

Nuts and edible seeds are also imperative and provide potassium, magnesium, vitamin E, and other antioxidants. High-fiber, low-sugar fruits such as kiwis, berries, rhubarb, and melon can also be included, up to ½ cup daily.

Grains and cereals that are very high in fiber and hence low in net carbohydrates should also be included. These include flaxseed, wheat bran, rice bran, corn bran, and oat bran.

The health-packed foods that supply essential nutrients such as vitamins, trace elements, antioxidants, and other phytochemicals can be incorporated easily into your daily diet. Start by thinking "vegetables and color." The greater the variety of color in your daily five servings of vegetables and low-carbohydrate fruits, the more likely it is that you will be including an assortment of beneficial foods.

We all get into certain habits that are hard to break, but some habits can be built upon in a positive way. For instance, most people have a salad sometime during the day. It's usually a side salad with lunch or dinner. It's also likely to be a rather bland and unimportant dose of iceberg lettuce.

Get creative and build a pharmafood salad by using healthier greens, like romaine lettuce or spinach. Then add color to it. How about dark green broccoli florets, red onion, chopped yellow peppers, and a sprinkle of sunflower seeds? Or lime green avocado and a small, chopped red tomato and yellow onions?

Now apply the same thinking to your current side vegetables. Remember when they were white potatoes and yellow corn? Now, start to think orange squash and medium green Brussels sprouts. Desserts used to be brown pastries, right? Try to think about red rhubarb and strawberry compote or fresh dark blueberries on yogurt. And don't forget to have a cup of green tea or a mug of great coffee or a small glass of red wine.

In the process of changing your mind-set to think about variety and color, you will be enhancing your health while moving toward a more appropriate weight. It's not as difficult as you might think. But you will have to work to familiarize yourself with the great variety of beneficial foods that are available.

What about adding a cup of homemade vegetable soup to your meal? Or even making it your whole meal? If you make your own soup, you can start with a can of premade vegetable broth (or make your own), add a can of diced tomatoes, and put in assorted vegetables that are in the kitchen — onions or leeks, zucchini or yellow squash, shredded kale or spinach. You're health-packing your diet, and you can bring the leftovers to work.

Another way to add assorted pharmafoods is to make sauces with vegetables and then put them over meats or fish. One idea is to make your own tomato-based sauce from diced tomatoes, chopped eggplant, peppers, and onions, flavored with garlic, basil, and oregano, simmered until your house smells like an Italian restaurant. Then add precooked chicken breasts and simmer until heated through.

Don't settle for a plain cheese or ham omelet when you can have a pharmafood omelet with sliced tomatoes, onions, and green peppers. Or how about one with chopped cooked spinach and onions with a little feta cheese?

See how easy it is? Use your imagination. Once you put your creative side to work, you will figure out more ways to fit these health-packed pharmafoods into your daily life. Your health will only benefit from your efforts.

SUMMING UP

AS A REVIEW, here are the guidelines you should follow as you embark on this diet:

1. Eat three meals a day, even if you don't feel hungry.
2. Don't count calories. Eat enough to feel satisfied but not enough to feel stuffed. You can eat as much as you like of the foods in Table 5.2 that don't indicate amounts.
3. Keep your net carbohydrate count at 15 grams per meal, 50 grams a day, or less. Remember, *subtract fiber from carbohydrates to get net carbs.*
4. Eat at least five servings of assorted vegetables every day, preferably from the other pharmafoods group. A serving is 1 cup of uncooked fresh vegetables or a half cup of cooked.
5. Make sure you choose foods from every corner every day.

Table 5.2 lists the foods in each of the four corners of the diet. The food items that are starred are ones that people with diabetes may have to be careful with.

Note that some foods are in more than one corner. For example, nuts have a lot of monounsaturated fat and they also have a lot of fiber.

TABLE 5.2
The Four Corners Diet

1. LOW-CARB FOODS

Unbreaded lean meats (remove external fat) including:	Cucumbers and unsweetened pickles
Beef	Green beans
Poultry	Pole beans
Pork	Wax beans
Veal	Mushrooms
Lamb	Okra
Game animals	Chinese vegetables
Tofu	Asparagus
Soybeans (limit ½ cup per day)	Celery
	Onions*
	Radishes
Fish, including canned in water or canola oil; look for ways to eat more fish	Tea, coffee
	Carbohydrate-free condiments (mustard, mayonnaise, vinegar, soy sauce; but avoid catsup)
All-meat sausages, hot dogs, and luncheon meats, in small quantities; eat only occasionally; low-saturated-fat choices are preferred	
	Butter (small amounts)
	Whole cream
	No-calorie gelatin
Shellfish	Egg-based custards and mousses*
Eggs	
Hard cheeses (except processed cheeses with added starches)	Artificial sweeteners
	Carbohydrate-free drinks
Soft brie-type cheeses	Sugar-free, carbohydrate-free syrups
Ricotta cheese*	Low-carb beer
Cottage cheese*	Dry wines (limit alcoholic beverages: one drink for women and two for men)
Cream cheese (plain)	
Melons*†	
Kiwi*†	Salt, pepper, spices

2. HIGH-MONOUNSATURATED FAT FOODS

Nuts and seeds (limit 4 ounces or ½ cup/day)
Avocados, guacamole
Olive oil
Canola oil
Unskinned poultry
Lean beef
Lean veal
Lean pork
Fish
Peanut butter

3. HIGH-FIBER FOODS

Nuts, sunflower and pumpkin seeds, and flaxseeds (limit 4 ounces or ½ cup/day)	Psyllium husks or powder; guar gum; xanthan gum
	Extremely high-fiber cereal* (net carbs must be not more than 10 grams per serving size)
Peanut butter	
High-fiber breads and crispbreads* where net carb count is less than 5 grams per slice (must limit to 2 slices/day)	Cabbage
	Tart apples*† and pears*†
	Okra
Spinach and other greens	Nopal
Bran (wheat, corn, rice, or oat*)	Eggplant

4. PHARMAFOODS

PROBIOTIC (at least 1 cup/day)	Nuts and edible seeds (limit 4 ounces or ½ cup/day)
Plain yogurt	Avocado
Plain kefir	Celery
Buttermilk	Onions and leeks
Soy yogurt	Garlic
	Soybeans
OTHER PHARMAFOODS	Peppers
All fresh or frozen, unsweetened berries†	Watermelon*†
Greens: kale, spinach, romaine lettuce, fennel	Cantaloupe*†
	Kiwi*†
All summer and winter* squashes	Salsa, tomatoes* (limit to ½ cup/day)
Cruciferous vegetables: broccoli, Brussels sprouts, cauliflower, cabbage, and sauerkraut	Beverages: tea, coffee, and dry wines (wine limit: one drink for women and two for men)

* Foods that people with diabetes may have to be careful about.

† Limit fruit to ½ cup a day.

There are some foods you will just have to forget about because they are so high in carbohydrates that even a small portion is a significant load. The no-nos include milk, potatoes, sweet potatoes, beets, turnips, rice, corn, peas, beans (except green, wax, pole, and soybeans), lentils, pasta, breads, bagels, cookies, cakes, most crackers, pretzels, and rice cakes. You'll probably miss them at first, but as you become accustomed to this new way of eating, you'll find that your interest in these high-carb foods will wane.

Table 5.2 is meant only as a guide, a starting place. As you become accustomed to the diet, you'll most likely find some new foods that fit the requirements of the various corners. Don't hesitate to use them. Be creative. Adapt the diet to your preferences. And *enjoy your food.*

▶ IF YOU HAVE DIABETES

IF YOU HAVE diabetes, you may have to be more careful with products like oat bran that, although they're high in fiber, may raise your blood sugar more than some others.

When you have diabetes, not only the carbohydrate count of a food, but also its *glycemic index value* is important. The glycemic index value tells you how quickly a food will raise your blood glucose levels. When you have type 2 diabetes, your pancreas may still have the ability to deal with carbohydrate loads that are released slowly into the bloodstream, so foods with low glycemic index values are better for you.

The Four Corners Diet does not focus on the glycemic index, but in general, highly processed foods like flour and bread have higher glycemic index values than high-fiber foods like vegetables. Almost no high-glycemic index foods are recommended when you're following the Four Corners Diet, so you shouldn't have to spend a lot of time learning about this. For you, more important than general glycemic numbers are your own personal glycemic index numbers—how quickly any particular food raises your *own* blood sugar levels. Use your meter to find out which foods are okay for you.

We've starred the problematic foods in Table 5.2. Winter squash may be a problem for you unless you restrict the amounts to 1/4 cup or less. Some people find they can eat some kinds of melon, and others cannot. As always, use your meter as a guide.

You may be surprised to see that cottage cheese is starred, because most people think of cottage cheese as a diet food. This is because the liquid in the cottage cheese may contain a lot of lactose, and cottage cheese raises blood glucose levels in many people. You can reduce the effect of the cheese by rinsing it in a colander.

Onions contain a lot of sugar, but they are also supposed to contain compounds that help with blood glucose control. In reasonable amounts they should be okay for you.

Yogurt, on the other hand, is a wonderful food for someone with diabetes, because it can be made into a yummy dessert, it gives you a lot of calcium, and—best of all—it has a very low glycemic index value and won't raise your blood sugar much at all. Kefir, of course, has the same benefits and some additional ones as well.

As noted, the bacteria in yogurt convert the sugar lactose into lactic acid. Lactic acid *can* be converted to glucose in the liver by a process known as gluconeogenesis. This is how the body deals with the lactic acid you produce when you exercise hard. However, this conversion is fairly slow, and when you're able to produce some insulin—just not an awful lot—your own pancreas may be able to deal with the slow release of glucose made from the lactic acid you eat. Again, use your meter and see how much yogurt you can eat without a significant effect on your blood glucose level.

If a cup is too much for you at one time, no problem. Just divide your daily cup into smaller portions and eat a little with each meal or snack. You could have a quarter cup of coffee-flavored yogurt for breakfast, a berry kefir shake with lunch, and a yogurt-cucumber salad with dinner.

You'll also want to be especially careful with the fat-free commercial yogurts you buy at the store. The added cornstarch and milk solids might be too much carbohydrate for you. If possible, make your own. It doesn't really take much work—and it's a lot cheaper.

When you have diabetes, soluble fiber is your friend. By slowing down the emptying of your stomach, soluble fiber slows down the rate at which glucose is taken up into your blood. Your handicapped pancreas may be able to deal with the slow, steady release of glucose instead of a sudden burst of glucose that you would get from a fiber-free meal.

Many traditional folk remedies for diabetes, such as nopal cactus, chia seed, barley, aloe, and fenugreek, are very high in soluble fiber.

If you buy psyllium powder, check the maltodextrin content. Maltodextrin is a carbohydrate derived from starch that is used as a filler. It has a very high glycemic index value. Some people can cope with small amounts of maltodextrin, so test before you decide. If possible, buy psyllium that doesn't contain maltodextrin. The boxes of pure psyllium you find in the drugstore are expensive. Look in health food stores for cheaper sources of psyllium powder as well as guar and xanthan gum.

Note that if you have the complication called gastroparesis, meaning slow and possibly sporadic emptying of your stomach, a lot of soluble fiber may not be a good idea.

Monounsaturated fat has also been shown to be beneficial for people with diabetes because it provides calories without raising your blood glucose levels and without affecting your insulin resistance, as saturated fat may do.

Pharmafoods of special interest for people with diabetes include cinnamon and Asian bitter melon (*Momordica charantia*).

SIX

Fitting the Four Corners into Your Lifestyle

EATING OUT

AMERICANS TODAY ARE busy. Because of this, you may be eating most of your meals in restaurants. This does make it more difficult to follow a healthy diet like the Four Corners Diet. Restaurants are in business to make money. Starches are cheap, and vegetables are expensive, so they'd rather fill you up with a plate that's mostly cheap pasta or rice covered in a sweetened, thickened sauce than to give you lean meats and fresh vegetables.

But if you're careful, you can follow the Four Corners principles even when dining out. Here are a few tips:

- ❖ Never order the soup unless it's beef, chicken, or vegetable consommé. No noodles, croutons, or crackers.
- ❖ Of course, no breads or pasta or potatoes or rice. If you order a burger, order it bunless or ask for extra pickles or

lettuce as a substitute. Ask for salad substitute or other vegetables or tomato slices instead of the potato or pasta side order. Don't let the waitress even leave bread or crackers at the table.

❖ Make your own salad dressing from oil and vinegar.

❖ Scrape off any breading and leave it on your bread plate.

❖ Ask for cheese and strawberries or strawberries and cream for dessert. You can sweeten it with the no-calorie sweetener on the table if you need to.

❖ Ask Chinese restaurants not to thicken your sauce with cornstarch or flour. It's better to have foods simply stir-fried without sauces.

❖ Remember that you can eat meat, chicken, fish, or eggs without any portion controls. But pile on the low-carbohydrate veggies and salads at every opportunity. Order extra sides of vegetables. And always trim excess fat.

These days more and more people are trying low-carb diets, and restaurants are responding to the need. So as time goes on, you will find more low-carb offerings on the menu. Just make sure to keep the other three corners in mind when you're ordering.

Even if you're not eating most of your meals out, you may be buying take-out food to bring home or zapping TV dinners for a quick meal after a hard day at work. Most of us have to use some convenience foods in order to have time to accomplish all the things we want to do. The trick is to make sure the convenience foods you eat are healthy ones.

Men, women, and children face different challenges in trying to eat healthy food in an unhealthy world. Following are some of the challenges each group faces.

WOMEN

WOMEN ARE THE traditional caretakers of the family. Even with the revolution in the workplace, with most households now having mothers who work, the business of planning meals and running the household has remained primarily women's work. Thus if you work outside the home, you may have resigned yourself to the fact that you're not superwoman and that it's okay to eat out or to bring home carry-out food.

Does this sound familiar to you? You've worked all day. It's five o'clock and you've got to do your grocery shopping, get home, and serve dinner before working on next morning's presentation or taking your kid to a meeting at school. You are in the supermarket with a list of healthy foods. Despite your best planning, it *still* takes a while to complete your shopping. Decision point. Do you go to the drive-up window and pick up burgers and fries? After all, you are exhausted by now. Your day isn't done yet. You've got all this to unpack and still another task or two to do. You could start the diet again next week, right?

Wrong.

What you need to do for situations like this is to have a plan ready before you ever get to this point. You need to establish new habits that are as convenient for you as the old ones were.

On the days when you have other things to do after work, make sure that dinner is started and cooking while you're doing your daily job. For example, have chili, stew, sausages and peppers, or a pot roast cooking in a slow cooker (crock pot). That way, all you need is a large salad and dinner's ready. Have chicken prepared and seasoned in a baking pan and show your son or daughter how to preheat the oven and throw it in an hour before you get home. Prior planning will reduce the chances of slipping back into old ways.

One thing that is so appealing about carry-out is that you can serve the food out of the cartons and throw away the mess. No cleanup. True, but if you stock your house with aluminum foil, cooking bags, and olive or canola oil spray (for the slow cooker and casserole pans), you can still keep cleanups to a minimum. Remember: if you have leftovers for dinner, you can take them for your lunch the next day and save money while you're improving your diet.

Chapter 8 gives more hints for how to reduce the amount of time you spend on shopping and cooking, as well as keeping your expenses down.

But let's say you haven't done any of these things yet and you're in that supermarket deciding whether to get carry-out or not. You still have another choice. Before you return to your old habits at the burger bar, head over to the deli section. Most markets have rotisserie chicken, turkey breasts, and pork roasts for sale. Buy one of these, pick up a bag of premade salad and a large bag of broccoli-cauliflower-carrot medley. While you are dressing the salad, you can steam or microwave the other vegetables. If you want, you can buy a jar of premade Alfredo, hollandaise, or cheese sauce (check for carb counts before you do to make sure the sauces aren't thickened with flour) and heat it up to put on the vegetables. The cost and convenience of that dinner rivals or beats the drive-through, yet gives you a real dinner. Splurge and buy some no-sugar-added ice cream for dessert.

Dieting can be a drag for women. Most diets deprive you of something you're accustomed to. We are not asking you to count calories or to eat funny foods. But we are asking you to adopt some new habits. Eventually, the market will catch up with the demand and we will have more appropriate and healthy high-fiber, high-MUFA, low–net carb convenience foods from which to choose. More and more are appearing on the shelves every day. Keep an eye out for them. Just make sure you're not substituting low-carb junk food for the high-carb junk food you've been eating. Fresh foods are always better than processed.

But for now, let's say you walked in the door and your kids attacked the bags looking for snacks. If you had the right things on your shopping list, they could pull out some high-fiber crispbread and tasty cheese spreads or peanut butter and start munching while you're getting dinner on the table. See, it's not so hard.

MEN

WHEN WE TRIED our diet out in a formal study (see Chapter 12), the men in the study thought we were kidding when we told them what was on the diet. Eat meat, fish, nuts, and cheese and have a glass of wine or a light beer? No problem. Just give up potatoes and rice and chips? You're kidding me. Eat more vegetables? And I'll lose weight? You're pulling my leg.

We had to tell them to try it to believe it.

Once they did try the plan, the men were the easiest to convince. They were also the most impressed with their weight loss, losing the "pooch" around the middle and the love handles they had carried for way too long and had accepted as middle-aged manhood. As the diet spread around, some of our most interesting testimonials came from men.

We heard many stories about the pride those men who lost weight felt when they ran into old buddies who hadn't seen them in a while. Their slimmed-down bodies and smaller waist sizes were quickly noticed and envied.

Why is this diet so good for men? One of the main reasons the diet was so well accepted by men is that it involved few changes for them. But those few changes had *large* impacts.

If you're like the men in our study, you aren't particularly interested in sweets. You get your excess carbohydrates from breads and potatoes. If we give you other vegetables, you'll accept them after a bit of coaxing. If you don't get pasta for dinner, so what? You'll be more than happy to eat roast chicken instead.

What may be more difficult for you is accepting the additional foods you need to make your diet nutritious. You'll have to eat more vegetables with a greater variety than you're probably accustomed to eating, and you'll have to increase monounsaturated fats and fiber and add fermented milk products to your diet.

Fortunately, most of the men in our study liked nuts and seeds, and olive oil was fine. Even yogurt or kefir was acceptable to the majority. The key is to have these around the house all the time.

Vegetables were another story. Some men really resisted eating vegetables. We found that this dislike for vegetables was lifelong. We could get them to eat sauerkraut, coleslaw, and green salad, but more than that and we encountered resistance.

Many men said, they were losing weight, so why did they have to eat more vegetables? In case you have the same question, we'll repeat the reasons for this. Almost everyone will lose weight on a low-carbohydrate diet, but unless the rest of the diet is followed as well, the results can be hazardous.

For example, up to 30 percent of people on one popular low-carbohydrate diet saw worsening of their lipid profiles, potentially increasing their cardiac risk. Following the Four Corners Diet in its entirety provides a safeguard against this occurring. That means increasing monounsaturated fats, increasing fiber, adding fermented milk products, *and eating a variety of vegetables, too.*

You may also have questions about alcohol. Studies have shown that small amounts of alcohol may have a positive health benefit. It doesn't mean that you *have* to drink, however. The Four Corners Diet provides an adequate amount of natural antioxidants in the other recommended foods. If you do drink, don't exceed the recommended amounts per day. That means one drink for women and up to two drinks for men per day. A drink is equivalent to one light beer, one five-ounce glass of dry wine, or one shot of whiskey or similar alcohol. That doesn't mean you can have more if you had none for the previous three days. Drinking more than recommended will raise your triglyceride levels and increase your cardiac risk in addition to the well-known social and other health impacts of excess drinking.

Men are often looked upon as the "grillmeisters" of their households. This diet is perfect for you to show your health consciousness and culinary expertise—and give the household's regular cook a welcome reprieve from cooking duties for the day. Use that grill as often as possible, with both direct and indirect cooking methods to ensure the best tasting meats, fish, and vegetables.

The only warning here concerns barbecue sauce, which is usually made with a lot of sugar. You'll have to experiment and make your own, or find sugar-free varieties. Perhaps you'll want to cultivate more smokiness or hot-spicy tastes in your cooking and fewer sugary flavorings. You can create a custom sauce to meet these goals and still be on the diet. If you're making a teriyaki marinade, you can easily substitute no-calorie brown-sugar sweetener into the recipe. Here's a chance to show off your creativity and create a unique sauce that's the best on the block instead of the ho-hum bottled stuff they use next door.

Make sure you have a variety of marinated vegetable salads in the refrigerator to serve with your grilled items. The Recipes section offers some good suggestions. Simple sliced cucumbers, onions, and green peppers in oil and vinegar make a great salad. Remember, if they're always waiting in the refrigerator, you won't have an excuse to substitute unhealthy choices.

CHILDREN

BOTH THE UNITED STATES and Europe are reporting a recent dramatic rise in the number of overweight and obese children, and this disturbing trend shows no signs of reversing. Worse yet, the incidence of type 2 diabetes and hypertension has been rising along with the trend in increasing weight. Abnormal, unhealthy lipid patterns are also being found in children with increasing frequency.

Children and adolescents can follow the general principles of the Four Corners Diet. The diet has been used in dozens of children with anecdotally reported success. We have informally studied the effects of this diet in a colleague's pediatric practice with moderately to severely obese preteens. The children lost weight. We found it useful to form a support group for the children and their parents at which both groups were able to share their successes and recipes.

It makes sense to start instilling good eating habits in our children now so they can avoid future problems with obesity. What kinds of things can we do?

- ❖ *Make sure you don't let your children persuade you to buy nonnutritious high-carbohydrate foods.* Children are under enormous marketing pressure to consume a variety of high-carbohydrate foods. Some common examples seen on television during children's programming include cereals made from refined flours; fruit-flavored, corn syrup–sweetened, starch-based snacks; high-starch fried or baked snacks; breakfast pastries made from refined sugars and milled flours (albeit "vitamin-enriched"); and ready-to-toast or microwave high-starch and/or high-sugar "hot" snacks.

  These items are compelling. They're often in large bright displays in the snack aisles of supermarkets and are often "features" at the end-of-aisle displays. The drinks that are sold to wash them down include highly sugared "juice" drinks and high-carbohydrate sodas, which are sold in increasingly larger sizes.

  You can't save everyone, but you can try to save your children. Teach them to ignore these displays. Make sure you don't keep such foods in the house. Keep tasty nutritious foods handy to offer when they need a treat. As your children get older, explain to them that these foods are designed to make a lot of money for their manufacturers, not to benefit their health, and let them learn to make good choices on their own.

- ❖ *Make nutritious lunches for your children to take to school, or do some research to find nearby stores that carry such foods.* Unfortunately, typical lunch and after-school hangouts are often fast-food restaurants and snack bars that tempt kids with high-carb French fries, candy bars, pop, and shakes. Your children will face not only the tempting high-carb foods, but peer pressure to eat what everyone else is eating.

  Thus they themselves will have to recognize the benefits of Four Corners eating and buy into it. They'll have to bring their own lunches or find stores at lunchtime in which to buy premade tuna, meat, and vegetable salads, cheese cubes, string cheese, hard-boiled eggs, hot vegetable and meat soups, and yogurt. And they'll need to wash them down with no-calorie pop, iced tea, or bottled water. This isn't impossible. It's just a new choice.

❖ *Help them find a buddy.* Children who are struggling with weight problems need to start eating right immediately. One of the best ways for them to change their eating patterns is to do it with a buddy. If they're not the only one with a meal from home or the only one who goes to the local market instead of the snack shop at lunch, it will be easier for them to change.

Surely they're not the only overweight kids in school. Ask your child if there's a classmate with a weight problem, one your child gets along with. Then speak with that child's parents to see if you could help them help their child follow the same diet.

In fact, finding a buddy is a good idea for adults, too. You are bucking the system right now, and it helps to have friends on your side. In your household, probably most of the members are sharing a problem with obesity. After all, you share the same genes and you're likely eating the same foods. Sometimes, the best diet buddies may be the other people in your own household. If you see this return to good eating as a family challenge, you may have more success. Try it.

❖ *Teach them how to make better choices at fast-food places.* What if all the kids are going to a pizza parlor? Can your children go? Of course, but teach them to order the thinnest-crust pizza. They put two pieces together and then discard the top crust. Bingo, they've just reduced the carbs by half. They should have a salad as well, with water or diet pop to drink.

What if everyone is going to a hamburger joint? What can your children eat? Teach them to order a double cheeseburger and discard most of the bun while eating. No fries. Diet pop or unsweetened or artificially sweetened iced tea. If they feel deprived, they can order a second double-cheese. This feeling of loss over the fries doesn't continue for long.

Kids will just have to avoid some fast-food places that offer no healthy options at all. You can figure out those places for yourself just by thinking of their menus. You also know what foods you simply cannot have in your household: none of those items listed at the beginning of this section, no candy, no high-carb snacks, no regular breads, no potatoes, no pasta, no rice.

Buy plenty of high-fiber crispbread, peanut butter, cream cheese, string cheese, nuts and seeds, tart apples, fresh berries, and plain yogurt (which you can sweeten with no-calorie sweetener and berries). You can use high-fiber, low-carbohydrate bread (with 3 grams of net carbohydrates and 8 grams of fiber per slice). There is also a low-net-carbohydrate, high-fiber tortilla shell on the market that is very useful for making tacos and quesadillas (all the fillings are okay). The count for that tortilla shell is 8 grams of fiber and 3 grams of net carbohydrates.

Children do have higher metabolic rates than adults. They're growing, of course. So, caloric intakes have to allow for this. You might think maybe they *could* cheat and get away with it. Unfortunately, this is not likely. If the cheating involves high-carbohydrate products, the results will be the same. It's better to allow children to eat to satiety with healthy foods. Once the high-carbohydrate (especially high-sugar-content) foods have been eliminated, children will eat the amounts of healthy food they need in order to grow.

One caveat for children: it is *very* important for overweight children to be checked out by their pediatrician before starting on a new diet. It is possible that your child has an endocrine problem. And if your child has been overweight for a while, he or she may have a medical complication of obesity already. The pediatrician can give the child a thorough checkup and order appropriate lab testing. Then if the pediatrician agrees, you can start the child on the Four Corners Diet.

▶ IF YOU HAVE DIABETES

IF YOU HAVE diabetes, your life is probably even busier than everyone else's. You not only have all the same problems everyone else has, but you've got to deal with your diabetes as well.

You're testing your blood glucose levels, sometimes many times a day. You have extra doctors' appointments. You have to run down to the hospital to get blood drawn for lab tests. The cold that is going around is just an inconvenience for most people. For you it causes a huge increase in your blood glucose levels, and you're worried.

You may think that taking extra time to fix whole foods and healthy meals is the last straw. Just remember that you also have more at stake here. The Four Corners Diet will help you keep your blood glucose levels under control in addition to helping you to lose weight if you need to lose—and most of us do. Keeping your blood glucose levels under control will help you to prevent complications. If you have very early signs of diabetes complications, keeping your blood glucose levels in the normal range may even help you reverse some of those complications, such as neuropathy or tingling of the hands or feet.

So it's really worth the extra bother. Your time is precious. But so is your health.

When you're eating out, one thing that helps is to learn to be assertive. Don't be embarrassed about explaining to the server that you have diabetes and can't eat sugars or starches. You may find that servers are more sympathetic and will go out of their way to help you choose something you can eat. Sometimes they'll even go out into the kitchen to ask the chef if the sauce on that chicken dish is thickened with flour. Or they'll let you substitute more green beans or salad for the mashed potatoes that come with the main dish.

One trick is to choose a couple of low-carb appetizers and a small salad instead of an entrée that's mostly pasta or rice.

Chinese restaurants are often the most difficult, because so many sauces are thickened with cornstarch. Japanese dishes tend to be high in sugar. Thai and Indian restaurants may offer a larger selection of things you can eat as long as you avoid the breads, noodles, and rice.

Be creative. At a restaurant known for its gooey desserts, one woman with diabetes asked for a second helping of a delicious zucchini Provençal dish instead of the dessert that came with the meal. Her dining companion, who wasn't diabetic, decided to do the same. The waitress came back and said everyone in the kitchen was laughing about the zucchini dessert at table 4, but both the diners were happy.

Once you get accustomed to being assertive and doing things a little differently than everyone else, dining out gets a lot easier.

SEVEN

My Kind of Food

AT THIS POINT you may be thinking, "Well, this does sound good. But how can I follow this diet when my family cuisine depends heavily on rice (or noodles, or potatoes)?"

The answer is, it's more difficult, but it's not impossible. The diversity of foods that can be prepared while staying within the recommendations of the Four Corners Diet is practically limitless. You just need to learn how to substitute for high-carbohydrate ingredients.

Furthermore, if, like most of us, you've become too dependent on convenience foods and take-out fast foods, you need to learn to replicate the convenience and "fast" aspects in your own home. While you're taking a hard look at your family's current food habits, you might take a deep look into your heritage and your family's recipe archives. You might be surprised at how healthy some of your grandparents' favorite recipes are.

Following are a few tips on making substitutions for the carbiest foods.

■

POTATOES

SOME OF YOU might not be able to envision life without potatoes. French fries will have to go. But cauliflower can make an amazingly good substitute for both mashed potatoes and potato salad.

One woman served her husband some mashed cauliflower without telling him what it was and, after eating everything on his plate, he said, "Pass the potatoes please." The Recipe section has a recipe for making what some people call "mashed fauxpotato."

For potato salad, just use your favorite recipe, but substitute cauliflower florets for the potato. Cook the cauliflower until it's just done, but not mushy. Cool and add florets to the other ingredients and dressing.

■

NOODLES

TODAY THERE ARE a variety of low-carb noodles available commercially. Reports on the taste range from "Blech. I'd rather eat cardboard" to "Tasted just like the real thing." If you want to go this route, look around until you find a brand that works for you.

Chinese bean thread, also called cellophane noodle, is made from mung beans, not wheat starch, and has more fiber and a much lower glycemic index value than regular pasta. Unfortunately, the fiber content isn't listed on the packages. Be careful to read the ingredients. Some brands add potato or other starches. This product does contain carbs, so you won't want to eat it every day. But for an occasional treat, a little bit is okay.

If you have access to a Japanese grocery store, look for shirataki noodles (konjac or konnyaku). They'll be packed in plastic in the refrigerator case. These noodles are made from the root of an Asian yam, and they're almost 100 percent fiber (glucomannan), so they're essentially free of net carbs, and you should be able to eat as much as you want.

The noodles *are* rather rubbery. In fact, they're used in Japanese stews because they don't get mushy when you boil them for a long time. But they take up sauces well when soaked before they are used. The glucomannan fiber is also supposed to help with lowering cholesterol. So these noodles are a good bargain, for your health.

Asian stores also often sell soy noodles in various shapes, including a wide noodle that could be used in a lasagna-type dish. They don't have the same texture as traditional wheat noodles, but they might be just what you need for certain recipes.

If you're really ambitious, you might want to try to make your own low-carb noodles from soy flour, eggs, and protein powder. Look for recipes in various low-carb cookbooks.

You can also substitute vegetables for some noodle dishes. For example, you can use vegetable spaghetti as a base for some pasta dishes. It's more watery, so you'll want to cut back on the liquid ingredients in the recipe.

You can use eggplant, Portobello mushrooms, or thinly sliced strips of zucchini instead of pasta in a lasagna-type dish. By doing so, you're also adding the beneficial fiber and vitamins from the vegetables.

Use finely shredded, lightly cooked cabbage in soups instead of noodles.

You can use sliced or chopped tofu as a macaroni substitute to make what some people call "macaphoni and cheese" or "mockaroni and cheese."

RICE

IT'S DIFFICULT TO replicate the special taste of rice, but our old friend cauliflower can be used to make a "pseudograin" that you can put your sauces on (see Recipe section). When served such a dish, one diner said, "What grain is this?"

The cauliflower "rice" makes an excellent substitute in dishes like fried rice because it absorbs the sauce nicely. It also works well in stir-fries.

BREADS AND MUFFINS

TODAY THERE ARE numerous brands of low-carb bread available commercially, as well as low-carb bread and muffin mixes. As with the noodles, look around until you find a brand that tastes good to you, preferably one that also contains a lot of fiber.

You can also make low-carb bread in a bread machine, or the old-fashioned way, using ingredients like soy flour, wheat gluten (not wheat gluten flour, which has more carbs), protein powder, ground flaxseed, wheat bran, and nuts.

Recipes for both breads and muffins abound both in low-carb cookbooks and on the Internet. A couple are included in the Recipe section.

■

PANCAKES

CREPE-STYLE PANCAKES are easy to make using soy flour or protein powder, eggs, and either water or cream. You can eat them with syrup or as wraps in place of sandwiches.

Heartier pancakes made with bran are also easy to make and are a great way to increase your intake of both types of fiber (see Recipe section).

■

STUFFING

YOU CAN MAKE stuffing by substituting pork rinds for the bread in the recipe. Or use low-carb bread. You can also simply add more of the non-bread ingredients to your favorite recipe, or add ground nuts.

■

TACOS

TACO SHELLS CAN be made from firm lettuce leaves. You can also microwave slices of cheese until they're hot. Shape into taco shapes and let cool. Or simply make a taco salad instead of tacos.

■

OTHER TIPS

USE PSYLLIUM, GUAR gum, xanthan gum, or a commercial product called NotStarch as a thickener instead of flour or cornstarch. The guar gum works especially well in place of cornstarch in thickening Chinese recipes because the resulting sauce is clear.

Use ground nuts, soy flour, or bran for breading.

In place of regular breadcrumbs, use low-carb bread or pulverized pork rinds.

Substitute grated zucchini, cauliflower, or a mixture of both for potatoes in your recipe for latkes. Remember, the real sour cream topping is allowed.

Use wheat bran or gums such as psyllium as a filler when making meatballs or meatloaf.

BE CREATIVE

YOU CAN PROBABLY invent some new low-carb recipes yourself starting from traditional recipes you've always used and making appropriate substitutions. Just remember to follow the guidelines of the Four Corners Diet. No more than 15 grams of carbs per meal or 50 grams per day. Eat something from each of the four corners every day.

It may be difficult to know exactly how much carbohydrate there is in "exotic" foods that don't list fiber counts. Some of these foods also won't be found in the U.S. Department of Agriculture's database.

After a while, you should have a good idea of which foods are dense with net carbohydrates and which ones are not. Meats, greens, and most above-ground vegetables (except corn and peas) don't have much starch. Grains and underground vegetables usually do.

If you'd rather stick to the tried and true, there are many low-carb cookbooks on the market today. If you have access to the Internet, there are also numerous low-carb sites that feature recipes, and even a low-carb-recipe mailing list that provides recipes almost every day as well as tips on coping with the low-carb lifestyle. Just avoid the recipes that are heavy in cream and butter—a lot of them are.

Make sure that your total meal, including the recipes you choose from these books and Internet sites, satisfies the requirements of the Four Corners Diet in addition to being low-carb. For your total health, cutting back on the carbs alone isn't enough. You need the nutrients from all four corners to optimize your health.

With a little creativity, the Four Corners Diet can be adapted to the cuisines of many nations.

Many Chinese recipes can be prepared using psyllium or guar gum to thicken the sauces instead of cornstarch. Dishes like whole steamed fish with vegetables would fit perfectly into the Four Corners Diet. Of course you'll have to give up the rice and noodles and congee.

Sweet Japanese sauces can be made with artificial sweeteners. Japanese shirataki noodles make a perfect Four Corners dish because they consist of 100 percent fiber. Again, you'll have to avoid the rice and noodles.

Italian food means more than pasta. A meal may consist of chicken, veal, or fish, large salads, and vegetables. You can use liberal amounts of Italian seasonings such as garlic, basil, and oregano, and reasonable amounts of cheese. Just go easy on tomatoes, which contain a lot of sugar.

Highly seasoned Latino chicken and pork dishes are fine for the Four Corners Diet. The fish and shellfish that are also often parts of this heritage are fine. You'll have to eliminate most rice and bean dishes, however. Black soybeans can be used in place of other types of beans.

Many Greek dishes go wonderfully with the Four Corners approach because Greeks use a lot of olive oil. You can make egg lemon soup without the rice. Greek salads are wonderful. Greek lamb and vegetable dishes are fine. Again, you'll have to omit the rice that is often part of a Greek meal.

Creole cooking is loaded with vegetables, fish, and shellfish. New Orleans omelets are legendary.

You can eat good French food if you choose carefully and avoid sauces, which are likely to be thickened with flour. The French often have cheese for dessert instead of sweets, which would be perfect for you.

Israeli and Arabic dishes include yogurt, salads, and fish, as well as healthy olive oil. But of course, you'll have to eliminate the rice that often goes along with them.

America is so diverse that most of us don't limit our menus to one national cuisine alone. If you pick the healthiest from all the cuisines, you'll have a varied as well as a healthy diet on the Four Corners plan.

▶ IF YOU HAVE DIABETES

IF YOU HAVE diabetes, you can use the tips described in this chapter to reduce your net carbohydrate intake, but you may have to be more careful of some of the "faster" carbohydrates, such as low-carb bread.

As always, use your meter as a guide. For example, some people with diabetes can eat bean thread with very little effect on their blood glucose levels. Others cannot. Test yourself one and two hours after a meal when you try a new food. Then test yourself again on another day.

Sometimes you'll find you'll be able to tolerate something like bean thread along with protein and fat for dinner, but you can't eat it by itself, especially early in the day. So test several times before you decide which of these foods will work for you.

Soluble fiber is particularly good for people with type 2 diabetes because it slows down the emptying of the stomach, which means the carbohydrate you eat won't get dumped into your system all at once, and your pancreas will be better able to cope. Thus a high-soluble-fiber food like shirataki is not only a substitute for pasta; it's also a type of pharmafood for you.

If you have gastroparesis (slow stomach emptying caused by damage to nerves from high blood sugar levels), however, you should be careful of foods that slow down stomach emptying even more.

EIGHT

Following the Four Corners Diet When Time and Money Are Scarce

B Y NOW YOU understand what kinds of foods are good for you. But you may be thinking: "I work all day. I don't have time for all that chopping and cooking," or "I can't afford to buy expensive lean meats and fresh vegetables year-round."

Yes, you can. The processed convenience foods that we Americans love to use are not only the most unhealthy foods. They're also the most expensive in terms of what you're getting for your money.

Manufacturers give you lots of cheap starches, unhealthy trans fats, cheap refined sugars like high-fructose corn syrup, cheap saturated fat, a lot of salt, artificial flavorings, artificial colorings, food additives to improve shelf life, and a little real food, put it into a fancy box, make it easy to reheat, and charge you a lot of money. Buyer beware.

Yes, those foods are convenient. But they're also expensive for the amount of food you're getting. And in the long run, they're even more expensive because they can damage your health, and the cost of fresh foods is trivial compared with the cost of health care.

What you need to learn as you adapt to this new way of eating is how to prepare nutritious weight-controlling foods without spending a lot of time or money. Following are a few tips to get you started:

❖ *Shop in quantity.* We can't all afford the time or expense it takes to shop every day for small quantities of fresh ingredients. But with a freezer, you can buy in bulk when the prices are good.

The items most frequently discounted in bulk are meats and seafood. These can easily be frozen in smaller quantities for later dinners. Nuts, edible seeds, flaxseed, and bran are also available in quantity discount from wholesale stores or directly from nut and seed companies. These can also be repackaged in smaller portion sizes and frozen.

You may not have thought of this before, but shopping for quantities at seasonal farmers' markets can be a great way to get fresh berries and cheeses. These are often organic as well. Buy berries by the case and, again, freeze in smaller packaging for later use. You'll often find the best buys in the autumn when frost has been predicted. The farmers want to get their produce sold before it's too late and are happy to sell large amounts at lowered prices.

❖ *Buy larger quantities of packaged, diet-friendly foods when they're on sale.* Sugar-free powdered beverages, diet soda, and sugar-free gelatins all can be stored for months.

❖ *Cook in bulk quantities and then freeze (or can, if appropriate) in smaller portion sizes for family dinners or single-serve lunches and snacks.* A favorite snack of seasoned, roasted chicken drumsticks is much easier if you bake a large panful and then freeze them. Individual drumsticks can be removed from the freezer and then microwaved for a quick snack. Make a large pot of soup or stew and then freeze a batch for a second meal at a future date.

❖ *Have plenty of single-serve containers available so you can put leftovers in them.* Then take leftovers from dinner to work for lunch the next day.

❖ *Freeze several single-serve portions to pop in the toaster.* When you make wheat bran waffles or high-fiber pancakes, multiply the recipe and cook them all at the same time. Then freeze the excess. You will have created your own toaster pop-ins—a great breakfast for those rushed mornings.

❖ *Make your own yogurt and kefir* from the recipes we have included in this book. It's much cheaper, and you can make quarts at a time for the cost of milk alone. You can also create yogurt cheese and spreads and dips on your own, saving the cost of processed foods.

❖ *Find your own treats.* You will save more money and be more likely to stay on the diet if you don't deny yourself your favorite "spoil-me" foods. Don't ever be caught without those good foods in the house. Buy fresh avocados and have an avocado salad. Toast nuts for ten minutes at 350°F to enhance their flavor and then sprinkle them liberally over your breakfast yogurt and berries. Grind toasted pecans and make pecan-crusted, pan-fried catfish fillets. Bake a big cheesecake (with a nut crust). You deserve it!

❖ *Grow your own—something.* If you have any space at all, including a patio pot, grow something edible. It may be mixed greens, cucumbers, green peppers—whatever you grow yourself will taste better and be cheaper than what you might buy. If you have no space for a garden, see if one of your friends does. Most home gardeners have too much produce in season and would be thrilled to sell it and happy to give it away.

Summary of Suggestions

SHOP and buy bulk fresh foods and meats.
FREEZE in smaller sizes (berries, nuts, seeds, bran, meats, seafood).
COOK in bulk quantities (soups, stews).
COOK double batches of toaster pop-ins (waffles, pancakes).
TAKE leftovers to work.
STORE in convenience sizes.
MAKE your own yogurt and kefir.
FIND your own treats.
GROW your own foods.

▶ IF YOU HAVE DIABETES

IF YOU HAVE diabetes, you've no doubt been told that it's important for you to get as much exercise as possible. One of the best forms of exercise for almost everyone—unless you have other medical problems that restrict your activity—is walking. If you so choose, you can walk on a treadmill at home or at an exercise club.

But wouldn't it be more fun for you to get your walking in while you're shopping for bargains in healthy food? Find a farmers' market and walk the whole periphery of the market at a good clip, glancing at the offerings, before you settle in for some serious shopping.

Carry the bulk bargains you've just purchased at the megastore to your car instead of getting someone to wheel them out for you. See if you can carry a few more pounds every time you shop. Then you'll know your muscles are getting stronger.

If you live in a city where there is more than one good grocery store in the same neighborhood, walk from one to another to check out the prices before you buy. Even if you're pressed for time, it won't take any more out of the day than walking on a treadmill or using an exercise bicycle for thirty minutes. And you'll be finding bargains at the same time.

If you live in the country, make sure you plant a garden or help a friend with a garden in exchange for some of the produce.

If you don't drive out to the country when the "pick your own" berry farms are producing. You'll get exercise along with big flats of berries to freeze for the winter.

Your time is precious. So combine your exercise with bargain hunting and you'll benefit twice.

NINE

Help! I'm Not Losing Weight

"**W**HY AM I not losing weight? I've followed the diet faithfully and I can't seem to lose. I think I've hit a plateau. Maybe this diet won't work for me."

We've heard this more than once. After a brisk four-pound weight loss in the first week, people are upset when they see no change in the scale the next week. Or they lose twelve pounds in the first month and then can't seem to move the scale at all for three weeks. Or they have a nice one- to two-pound weight loss every week for three months and then mysteriously stop when they still have several pounds to go. Do these things mean diet failure? Are they unusual? No, there are many reasons for the start-and-stop behavior on the diet.

First, plateaus are common. You didn't put the weight on evenly and nonstop, and you won't take it off evenly and nonstop. These plateaus are your body catching its breath. Sometimes plateaus last a week, sometimes a month. Don't let these little bumps throw you off the straight and narrow path to a slimmer you. Relax and let your body take you there. It *will* happen.

One of the worst things you can do while dieting (and of course we all do it) is to weigh yourself at every opportunity whenever you're near a bathroom scale. It's amazing that your weight can vary so much over the course of a day. But weight changes during the day don't mean you've gained or lost fat. A rapid change in weight from day to day is just water retention and loss. It takes about 3,500 calories to gain or lose a pound of fat. So a three-pound loss in one day is usually just a water shift, because you certainly cannot burn off 10,500 calories in one day unless you're running a marathon!

Women sometimes hold on to water at various times of the month, so keep that in mind if you're a woman of childbearing age.

The best reflection of fat loss is your waist measurement, preferably measured at the same time of day, and not right after a meal. That doesn't change minute to minute.

One common reason for a slow weight loss is a drug interference. Many drugs induce stress hormones that counteract the mechanisms we are trying to induce with the Four Corners Diet. Steroid drugs are the biggest culprits, followed by nonsteroidal anti-inflammatory drugs including aspirin and ibuprofen; estrogens such as birth control pills and hormone-replacement therapies; blood pressure medications; and antidepressants.

However, even if such drugs can slow down weight loss, *do not stop taking any drug without your physician's guidance.* Your doctor has prescribed these drugs for a medical reason, and you should follow your physician's advice. The diet may still work for you, but just at a slower rate. So please be patient.

A sluggish thyroid gland can also slow things down. If you have not been tested for hypothyroidism in the past year, ask your doctor to check this out with a blood test called the *thyroid-stimulating hormone*—often shortened to TSH—test. Sometimes, a perfectly normal thyroid gland can become sluggish because of a lack of iodine in the diet. We suggest that you always use iodized salt to maintain a plentiful supply of iodine.

Not eating enough can also slow weight loss to a crawl. It's hard to believe, but it's true. If your body senses that it's not getting enough calories, it thinks it's starving, so it tries to conserve calories by *slowing your metabolism down.* That also slows down your weight loss. So *do not* skip meals or try to reduce calories to try to speed up your weight loss. It just won't work long term; instead, it will actually work against you.

Hidden carbohydrates are another weight-loss trap. You think you're eating less than 50 grams per day, but you forgot to count the 1 gram per packet of sweetener and you use ten packets per day. Don't forget to look at *all* labels and count *every* source of carbohydrates. For example, even black coffee contains a few carbs (about 0.8 grams per cup). Don't trust food labels alone. Make sure they agree with your carbohydrate counter book. Always assume the worst case.

Food sensitivities can affect some people. Examples are caffeine, citric acid in soft drinks, nuts, dairy products like cheese, and red meat. Different strokes for different folks. Try cutting certain foods out of your diet to see if it helps.

And finally, alas, there are a few individuals who will not lose weight on this diet. We don't know why. Maybe we missed something in counting the carbohydrates. Maybe the hyperinsulinemia is not easily shut off and even our reduced carbohydrate limits are too high, so the limited carbohydrates end up turned into fat stores in these people.

However, don't think you are one of these people until you've given the diet a truly fair chance of about six months. We had one overweight woman who lost only seven pounds in the first three months but felt so much better on the diet that she stuck it out. She had lost twenty-five pounds at the end of a year. That probably doesn't sound like much to some folks until you realize that this was the first time in her life she had *ever* lost *any* weight, no matter what she had tried, including liquid low-calorie diet fasts. That twenty-five-pound weight loss plus her feeling of well-being and great energy made her feel like a million dollars.

Finally, your body will not just keep losing weight. The Four Corners Diet will not make you disappear or turn you into a pin-thin fashion model. For the first few weeks you may lose two to three pounds per week. Then your loss will slow to one to two pounds per week for a few months, then down to one pound per week, then one pound per two to three weeks. Eventually your body will find the level it wants to stay at, which should be close to your ideal weight. If you were very overweight, this loss will continue until you have reduced many pounds and several belt sizes. But if you were only a few pounds overweight, your weight loss may subside in as little as two to three months. And, if you are absolutely normal weight (and normal BMI) and have chosen to follow this diet for hypoglycemia or high triglycerides or known hyperinsulinemia, remember that these conditions may improve with no weight loss at all.

If you're not losing weight because you fall off the wagon and cheat,

don't get angry with yourself. Old habits are hard to break.
self in the mirror and say the following to your image. Say
so you can hear it: "Are you serious about losing weight? T
this to happen again. You are not a child. Grow up and tak
for yourself. There was no reason to eat that unhealthy junk

Then get right back on the diet at the point you left off. Y   . . nave
to go through the first phase again. You still have your fat-burning
enzymes. It will take your body two or three days to recover from the carbohydrate shock, but then you'll be back in the saddle again.

However, if you break the diet for more than two meals, you will have
to start at square one again. Later, when you have lost most of your
weight, you will find the same holds true for diet vacations. For example,
if you visit a country that is famous for a particular dish, try it once, and
then get right back on the diet. Your body will always forgive these little
indiscretions so long as you remain in control.

If ever you feel you are losing control, *immediately return to the Phase
1 transition diet*. You should soon be back on track again.

Just remember, if you're not losing pounds every week, don't give up.
Know what's happening to your body. Keep the faith. And keep the diet.

▶ IF YOU HAVE DIABETES

IF YOU HAVE diabetes, you may have two strikes against you when it
comes to losing weight. First, type 2 diabetes is associated with what
some people call *thrifty genes,* meaning that you gain weight very easily
and lose it very slowly. If you've been overweight since you were a child,
even when you were eating a healthy diet or eating exactly the same
amount of food—maybe even less—than your skinny friends, then you
probably have thrifty genes.

If you come from a culture that until very recently was exposed to
cycles of feasting and fasting, for example, an agricultural culture in a
part of the world subject to periodic droughts and famines, then it's
even more likely that you have thrifty genes. Your ancestors who were
able to store fat easily during the short periods of plenty probably survived when their skinny friends perished, because they were able to live
off their fat in the famine years.

Now, however, in a society of abundance, those thrifty genes can be
a liability. It makes it more difficult for you to lose weight. The thing to

keep in mind is that it's not your fault that you inherited those genes. Life is very unfair, and you got a bad break in that area.

But just because it's unfair doesn't mean you should accept your fate (and fat) and make no effort to change. Sticking to the Four Corners Diet will help you control your hunger. When you have type 2 diabetes, you have higher blood glucose spikes after carbohydrate-containing meals than people without diabetes. When your blood glucose level begins to come down rapidly, you may find that you are ravenously hungry. The Four Corners Diet will even out these spikes and reduce your hunger, as well as improve your overall blood glucose levels. And near-normal blood glucose levels mean greatly reduced chances of diabetic complications.

A second strike you have against you in your efforts to lose weight is the medications you may be taking to help control your blood glucose levels. Some of these medications, including the sulfonylurea drugs, the glitazone drugs Avandia and Actos, and insulin itself, contribute to weight gain in some people. Metformin, on the other hand, does not cause weight gain and even helps with weight loss in some people.

So if your doctor prescribes one of these drugs and tells you to lose weight, but you gain weight instead, even on this diet, see your doctor again and discuss whether perhaps another drug would work just as well for you.

If you're trying your hardest and the weight doesn't come off easily, don't blame yourself—and don't let your health care people blame you, either. Your difficulty losing weight is probably not your fault.

TEN

Keeping the Weight Off

I F YOU'VE EVER lost weight before, you know it's a lot easier to lose weight than it is to keep it off. You can lose weight on almost any kind of diet. The problem is, if the diet is too restrictive, you'll eventually abandon it, revert to your old eating patterns—the ones that made you gain weight in the first place—and put the pounds back on . . . with interest.

"It wasn't unusual for me to lose and gain thirty or forty pounds a year."

"I've lost and gained over two hundred pounds in my lifetime. I've tried every diet that's been out. I've never stayed where I want to be."

Could this be you? If you've now lost the weight you wanted to lose, you don't want to get caught in this yo-yo diet trap. So how can you make sure the Four Corners Diet becomes your permanent way of eating, your way of life?

One thing people who have succeeded in keeping the weight

off share is a total change in the way they look at foods, so the change becomes permanent, as does the weight loss.

"The life change came as I learned to live without all the extra sugar that has been added to all the foods and condiments and sauces that we eat," said Dr. Berry L., who was mentioned in Chapter 1. He is one of the original followers of the Four Corners Diet and has been following this way of eating for the past six years. After one year on the diet, he'd lost seventy-five pounds and twelve inches of fat from his waist.

This personal commitment to healthy eating persists today—as does the weight loss. He continues to eat foods that maintain his health and his weight. He's a discriminating shopper. He reads labels on everything. He's particular about what he eats. He's made a real "life change."

The Four Corners approach to eating has also been successful with young people. "I just won't eat anything that could hurt me again," said Mike O., a college student who'd gained enough weight during the first two years of college to be told by his doctor that he'd have to start taking blood pressure pills for his newly diagnosed hypertension. He decided to try our diet first.

Mike O. lost eighty-five pounds in a year, and in the process he also lost his diagnosis of hypertension. That was two years ago. Today, he's a discriminating eater who's managed to find restaurants that allow *you* to choose the foods you eat—no automatic side orders of high-starch, high-sugar foods. He's refined his willpower to look past the temptations that surround us—the supersized fries and oversized sugar-filled beverages. His former diet of fast foods—no vegetables except potatoes; vending-machine snacks; high-sugar desserts—had literally sickened him. Paying attention is what's keeping him healthy now.

We have seen many other successful dieters who have managed to maintain their weight loss. Most of the people who currently follow this way of eating have had problems with weight their entire lives. They've lived with the restrictions imposed by other diets and have lost weight in the past, but it always came back. But this time it's different. By observing their success, we have come up with a few suggestions that will help you do the same.

❖ First, make it your family's diet, not just your own. If you have to constantly create multiple meal plans, you'll get tired eventually and revert to "everyone else's diet." This diet is healthy, and it will be good for your family as well as for you.

❖ Second, don't think of it as a "weight loss diet" that is a temporary, restrictive thing. Everyone is on some sort of diet. What you put into your mouth is your diet, and it can be healthy or unhealthy. Think of the Four Corners Diet as the way you meet your nutritional needs and keep yourself healthy, a healthy way of eating. You want to eat a balanced diet that is low in saturated fat, high in good fats, low in unneeded starches and sugars, and high in healthy fiber, vitamins, and pharmafoods.

❖ Third, diversify your recipe collection. Get new, healthier ideas. Scan the Internet. Ask your friends. Talk and read about food. Don't feel guilty when you eat. Eat slowly and *enjoy your food.*

❖ Fourth, become an expert on your own. There's so much information developing about the health benefits of foods. Who'd have thought we'd find out that certain foods can enhance your immunity, make you less prone to heart disease, lower your blood pressure, and protect you against some forms of cancer? That's what you should be eating, right? Right. Once you realize that some foods work to promote health while others might worsen or even cause health problems, it'll be mighty hard to eat those bad foods, won't it?

As Phil G. said in Chapter 1, "This is not a diet, it's a way of life." Don't ever go back to the unhealthy diet you were on before. Like Mike O., resolve never again to eat anything that will hurt you. When your new way of life becomes permanent, your weight loss will be permanent as well.

▶ IF YOU HAVE DIABETES

IN SOME WAYS, having diabetes is an advantage when it comes to sticking with a diet for the long term. At the present time, diabetes is not curable. However, it is controllable. You know that one of the essential factors in that control is your diet. And you should have the advantage of owning a blood glucose meter to help you stay on track.

People without diabetes may be tempted to try some high-starch foods occasionally, on the theory that "one day off the diet out of three hundred and sixty-five won't hurt me." Then there's the danger that 1 day turns into 3 and then 7 and eventually 365, and all the benefits of the new, healthy way of eating are lost and the weight comes back.

But when you have diabetes, those high-starch foods will make your blood glucose levels soar. You can see the results on your meter. Your vision may get blurry. You may feel tired. You may even feel pain or tingling in your feet. Was that starchy food really worth it? Most people decide it's not.

So be happy that you've found a way of eating that lets you eat a wide variety of healthy foods that fill you up, so you're not hungry. And use your meter as a guide. If your blood glucose goes up a lot after a new food, don't eat that food again. Or eat a much smaller portion. Your meter is your friend.

ELEVEN

Type 2 Diabetes

I F YOU HAVE type 2 diabetes, you've probably already learned a little bit about it. But it never hurts to review.

Type 2 diabetes is—by definition—caused by insulin resistance. Insulin resistance also causes a related condition called insulin resistance syndrome (also called metabolic syndrome or syndrome X), which is described in Chapter 13. You remember that having insulin resistance means that, for some reason that no one really understands completely yet, even when you are able to produce plenty of insulin, that insulin isn't as effective as it should be, especially in the muscle cells.

Because muscle cells need insulin to help them take glucose out of the blood, when you have insulin resistance, your blood sugar tends to be higher than it should be. Your pancreas senses that and produces even more insulin than normal. Thus you become hyperinsulinemic, meaning you have high levels of insulin in the blood.

So what's the difference between insulin resistance syndrome and type 2 diabetes? The crucial factor here is the beta cells in your pancreas, the specialized cells that produce insulin in response to demand. Some people's beta cells have no problem producing the huge amounts of insulin that are required when you have insulin resistance. People who have strong beta cells like that never get diabetes, no matter how much weight they gain and how much insulin resistance they have. However, they are hyperinsulinemic and are at greatly increased risk of heart disease.

If you have diabetes, you have genes that—again for reasons no one really understands yet—seem to "burn out" when required to produce supernormal amounts of insulin. At first they're able to produce enough to overcome the insulin resistance. Then, especially if the insulin resistance increases, they can't cope with the increased demand. They start to fail. Your blood glucose levels start to climb.

Increased blood glucose levels are toxic to beta cells. This is called glucotoxicity. So the beta cells burn out even faster, producing less and less insulin and eventually allowing your blood glucose levels to rise so high that someone notices and tells you that you're diabetic.

Thus type 2 diabetes is what some call a two-hit disease. In order to get it you need both insulin resistance and beta cell genes that can't cope with the increased demand.

In the early stages of the disease, your blood glucose levels may go too high only after you eat a meal containing carbohydrates. In later stages, even your fasting blood glucose levels will be abnormally high.

When you have diabetes, you can't produce enough insulin to keep your blood glucose levels normal, especially after you eat carbohydrate foods. So why, you may wonder, do many physicians and dietitians tell people to eat a lot of carbohydrate foods? Why does the American Diabetes Association (ADA) diet tell people with diabetes to "make starches the star"? Why do dietitians tell people with diabetes to put raisins in their oatmeal and bread crumbs in their meatloaf to "get the carb counts up"?

To answer this question we have to go back a bit and look at the history of diabetic diets. Years ago, before anyone knew what caused diabetes, some people told those with the disease to eat a lot of starches, even candy. Their logic was that the patients were losing a lot of sugar in their urine, so it was important to replace that sugar by eating even more.

Others supported low-carbohydrate diets. One diet proposed in 1797 said people with diabetes should eat only blood pudding and old rancid meats.

Type 2 Diabetes

In the early 1900s, just before the discovery of insulin, a standard diabetic diet was a very low-carbohydrate diet that was similar to low-carbohydrate diets today. It helped people with type 2 diabetes keep their blood sugars down. It—and a real starvation diet when the low-carbohydrate diet wasn't enough—also helped people with type 1 diabetes, who produce no insulin at all, stay alive longer. But no diet was able to keep them alive for very long, and type 1 diabetes was always fatal.

Then in the 1920s, insulin was discovered, and some people thought that diabetes had been cured. People with type 1 diabetes who looked like walking skeletons and were close to death started regaining weight. They started living lives that were close to normal. However, most of them continued to follow the then-standard low-carbohydrate, high-fat diets of the time.

Although the type 1 diabetic children survived childhood and grew into adults, many of them eventually died of heart disease at a relatively young age. In the 1950s, attention was being paid to studies that showed that heart disease rates were increased in people who ate high–saturated fat diets. Hence in 1979, it was decided to reduce the amount of fat in the diet of people with type 1 diabetes and to increase the carbohydrate content to 55 to 60 percent of total calories, also increasing the amount of insulin they injected to cover the extra carbohydrates they ate.

Eight years later, because people with type 2 diabetes also usually die from heart disease, these recommendations were made for people with type 2 diabetes as well, even though most of them weren't able to cover the extra carbohydrate with insulin. At the time, it was believed that the high blood glucose levels they had after such meals weren't harmful. In fact, there were no studies showing that high blood glucose levels caused the many complications of both types of diabetes, and doctors were more worried about having their patients avoid low-blood-sugar reactions than having blood sugar levels that were too high.

During this period, studies showed that a high-carbohydrate-*and-fiber* diet resulted in lower insulin resistance and lower postprandial blood glucose levels than the standard American diet or the high-glycemic-index ADA exchange diet, which doesn't tell you what kind of carbohydrate you should eat as long as you eat the amount specified in the diet.

Finally, in 1994, the ADA decided that perhaps a high-carbohydrate diet wasn't best for everyone with type 2 diabetes and suggested individualizing diabetic diets and sometimes substituting monounsaturated fat for some of the carbohydrates.

Unfortunately, some physicians and dietitians don't seem to have gotten the word and continue to prescribe lots of starches to all their patients.

Some dietitians also seem to have forgotten that the original studies emphasized high-fiber carbohydrates and thus urge their clients to eat a lot of breakfast cereals, sweet fruits, bread, and rice, all foods that cause a rapid increase in blood glucose levels.

People also seem to have forgotten that the famous Seven Countries study showing a relationship between fat intake and heart disease rates focused on countries that ate high amounts of saturated fat. In Greece, where people ate a lot of monounsaturated olive oil, rates of heart disease were low. You should also remember that the populations that ate a lot of saturated fat were also eating a lot of carbohydrates at the same time.

Thus studies suggesting that the best diet would be high in fiber and monounsaturated fat became misinterpreted to mean that the best diet would be high in starch and low in all kinds of fat.

The Four Corners Diet is an approach that should overcome these problems and misinterpretations. It will help you lose weight. Losing weight will help reduce your insulin resistance. Some insulin resistance is genetic, and there's nothing much you can do about that. But being overweight increases your insulin resistance. No one is certain why, but some chemical messengers—including tumor necrosis factor-α the newly discovered resistin, and most likely other factors that have not yet been discovered—are secreted by fat cells when the fat cells get full, and these substances increase insulin resistance.

But the low-carbohydrate part of the diet will also have a tremendous impact on your blood glucose levels. If you have type 2 diabetes and are not taking insulin or sulfonylurea drugs, your blood sugar levels will be much lower at all times than they would be if you were on a high-carbohydrate diet.

In recent years the results of a landmark study, the Diabetes Control and Complications Trial, known as the DCCT, showed without a doubt that people with type 1 diabetes who kept "tight control," meaning their blood sugar levels were lower, on average, had fewer diabetic complications. Later a British study and a Japanese study showed the same thing in people with type 2 diabetes.

Even more recently, studies have shown that two-hour postprandial blood sugar levels are the best predictors of future problems. People with lower levels had fewer cardiac deaths. The old days, when they said postprandial levels don't matter, are gone.

If you have type 1 diabetes or have type 2 diabetes and are taking insulin shots, of course you can cover any carbohydrates with insulin. However, it is very difficult to mimic by insulin injections the exquisite control of blood sugar levels that occurs in nondiabetic people. Your injections have to match your intake exactly, accounting for other factors such as exercise, stress, and the rate at which your stomach empties. When you eat a lot of carbohydrates, you're more likely to "roller coaster" from highs to lows back to highs again. Limiting your carbohydrate intake will smooth out these peaks and valleys.

Keeping your blood glucose levels close to normal is the best possible thing you can do to prevent diabetic complications like blindness, kidney failure, and amputation of your legs. Keeping blood glucose levels close to normal will have a positive effect on your cardiac risks, too, although the effect is not as great. Hence you need to monitor your lipid levels and blood pressure as well and add medication for those conditions if warranted.

This diet should improve your lipid levels. And weight loss should improve your blood pressure levels. Overall, your cardiac risk factors should improve.

However, we are all individuals, with individual physiologies. Most people with type 2 diabetes do well on a diet like this. There are always exceptions. Some people find that fat of any kind, even monounsaturated fat, causes problems for them and that they can control their blood glucose levels better on a high-fiber, low-fat diet.

We care about your overall health. So we urge you to try this diet, but to simultaneously monitor your blood glucose levels, your lipid levels, your blood pressure, and any other parameters your doctor thinks are important for you. Then, after a few months, take a look at the results and see if this diet is the best for you. If you think you would do better on a low-fat diet, try that for a few months, monitor your lab results, and then decide.

If you do decide to switch to a low-fat diet, you'll still be better off if you follow most of the principles of the Four Corners Diet. Try to make what little fat you do eat the healthy monounsaturated kind. Eat a lot of fiber. Eat probiotics and pharmafoods. Avoid fast-acting sugars and starches. Avoid processed foods. Eat as many of your carbohydrates as possible in the form of high-fiber vegetables.

Stay healthy—and enjoy your food.

TWELVE

Science:
Our Studies

■

WEIGHT-LOSS STUDY

ANY DIET CAN sound good on paper. But we didn't want to publicize our diet until we were certain it was safe. Hence in 1998 we conducted a twelve-week research study of the then-named Goldberg-O'Mara diet in moderately to severely obese subjects. This research project was conducted at a major Chicago hospital and was approved by its institutional review board, the committee that monitors research on human subjects.

We asked thirty volunteers to participate in the formal study of the diet. To qualify, they had to be obese, with a BMI greater than 29, have normal thyroid gland function, and not be under a physician's care for treatment of diabetes or other serious medical conditions for which they were on medication. Several volunteers who were hypertensive (had high blood pressure) joined the study with their doctor's written permission. Here's what they did.

The participants were told to eat their usual excess of carbohydrates for three days and then come to the laboratory for a fasting five-hour glucose tolerance test. For this test, they came to the lab at 8 A.M., having had nothing to eat since 7 P.M. on the previous evening. The laboratory phlebotomist (the technician who draws your blood) measured their height and weight and then drew two tubes of blood from their arms. Those blood samples were obtained to screen the volunteers for fasting blood sugar levels in addition to thyroid tests and a host of other tests that checked for abnormalities of liver and kidney function, blood lipids, and other markers of nutritional status.

Then we started the glucose tolerance test. Each person was given a flavored glucose drink containing 75 grams of carbohydrate, to be completely consumed within ten minutes. From that point on, they stayed calm and remained sitting in the reception area without smoking, eating, or drinking. Each hour on the hour, for the next five hours, another tube of blood was drawn.

The first two hours of this test are usually relatively easy for the people being tested. If you have a normal metabolism, the whole test should proceed without incident. However, obese people do not have a normal metabolism, and we found that certain things started to happen around three to four hours into the test. Some people felt nauseated; others got chills, sweats, or palpitations. In any case, most of our obese subjects did not feel well. By five hours, however, everything was back to normal for most of the volunteers, and after the last tube of blood was drawn, they rushed down to the cafeteria for a late combination breakfast, lunch, and snack.

Meanwhile, the blood tubes were sent to the laboratory for analysis. Each of the glucose tolerance blood samples was analyzed for levels of both glucose and the hormone insulin.

Once the entire battery of tests was completed and the results were reviewed by us, the volunteers were asked to start the diet. They were told to maintain a detailed diary of their food intake and to return each week for a weigh-in and nutritional counseling.

Initial Lab Results

It was no surprise to us that 75 percent of the overweight volunteers had a high fasting insulin level compared with the fasting insulin levels of people with a BMI of less than 25. However, almost 90 percent had very high (greater than 50 milliunits per liter [360 picomols per liter]) insulin levels at one and two hours after drinking the glucose solution. Most overweight people are insulin resistant. Their muscle cells "resist" the actions of insulin. So in order to keep their blood glucose levels normal, they must put out much more insulin than a normal-weight person needs. This same insulin resistance is found in people with type 2 diabetes (see Chapter 11). Type 2 diabetes and obesity are kissing cousins.

Other test results were unremarkable. Most subjects had cholesterol values in the "desirable" range (less than 200 milligrams per deciliter [mg/dL]) and high-normal triglyceride levels (less than 200 mg/dL). There were a few exceptions. One volunteer had triglyceride levels over 800 mg/dL. A few had mild elevations in the serum enzymes that can indicate liver problems. None had high uric acid levels, an indicator of gout and also often associated with the metabolic syndrome described in Chapter 13. All had normal kidney function test results.

Into the Diet

At the weekly sessions, the volunteers were weighed and we reviewed their diet diary. If we felt they needed to modify their food intake, we suggested different food choices. Interestingly, one of the main problems we found at the beginning of the diet was that the participants didn't eat enough. We told you about this phenomenon before. People badly want to lose weight and often will try to starve themselves or skip meals in order to accomplish some weight loss. They were so used to trying low-calorie diets that they were afraid to eat. Even though we had explained it to them, they couldn't believe that *this diet doesn't work that way.*

However, we quickly reassured them and made sure they had adequate food intake to prevent their bodies from slowing their metabolism down because of inadequate calories. Their usual caloric intake was about 2,000 to 2,200 calories.

Another common finding was a lack of fiber in the diet, which led to constipation. We emphasized that after the transition time, they had to eat at least five servings a day of high-fiber, low-starch vegetables and reinforced the idea of eating fermented milk products such as kefir, buttermilk, or yogurt daily. This was new to most of the volunteers. They were not accustomed to eating that many vegetables and that large a variety and were unaccustomed to fermented milk products.

We probably shouldn't have been surprised, knowing the usual eating habits of Americans. There seems to be so much stress placed on eating the high-carbohydrate cereals, pasta, and breads at the base of the USDA Food Pyramid that many consumers have forgotten about vegetables— despite the current mantra of nutritionists to "eat more fruits and vegetables." Most people ignore that advice and continue to eat burgers and fries. Those who do remember the nutritionists' advice tend to remember the fruits and forget the vegetables, drink more low-fiber orange juice or sweetened fruit drinks, use more sweetened ketchup, and leave the broccoli and spinach at the store.

We found that many of our volunteers did not cook at home. They ate most or all of their meals in the hospital cafeteria or at restaurants. This made it difficult for them to supplement with wheat bran and other fiber. We suggested that they eat a 100 percent wheat bran cereal with artificially sweetened kefir for breakfast, counting the net carbohydrates to keep within the 12- to 15-gram net carbohydrate per meal allowance.

Psyllium husk fiber is an excellent dietary supplement to prevent constipation and to lower cholesterol levels. Most people don't like to drink the commercial products. However, we suggested that the fiber be added to pancakes, meatballs, or even protein shakes for breakfast.

Our diet called for eating lots of nuts and seeds to enhance the intake of monounsaturated fats. This was well accepted by the group. They generally liked nuts and edible seeds but had been avoiding them because of a misconception regarding their high fat content. We explained that nuts have mostly good fats. Once they understood this, nuts became a mainstay dietary addition.

Eating nuts had a side benefit of preventing the potassium and magnesium imbalances that are common with other low-carbohydrate diets. One of the symptoms of a magnesium imbalance is severe night cramps in the calf muscles. None of our volunteers experienced this problem.

Three of the volunteers did not return for the first weigh-in and did not return our telephone calls. Maybe they just wanted all the free lab work. Maybe they couldn't get through the transition phase. We don't know. During the remainder of the study, we lost three more participants. One got sick and her physician insisted that she stop the diet; one got severe diarrhea and thought it was due to the diet; and the third couldn't give up beer and dropped out after three weeks.

That left twenty-four people who completed the entire twelve weeks of the study. That's an 80 percent compliance rate. As you read in Chapter

2, most dieters give up on their diets. Why then did 80 percent of the volunteers stick with this diet? Is it because the diet works with no feelings of deprivation? Perhaps it is because the weight came off so easily, together with an overall feeling of well-being. We're not certain what caused this feeling of increased well-being. It could be related to the production of ketones on a low-carb diet (see Chapter 13). Whatever the reasons, a diet that retains 80 percent of its subjects has to be doing something right.

Unlimited Energy

The other great benefit of the diet reported by all the research subjects was their increased energy levels. No more afternoon "crashes." No more crawling home after work and falling asleep in the chair after dinner. This diet gives something that no low-calorie or low-fat diet can provide. It provides an unlimited source of energy. You will have to experience it yourself in order to believe that dietary modifications alone can produce such a dramatic change in your alertness and mood.

One of our research volunteers told us that she looked forward to doing housework when she got home. She felt so good that she even brushed off the fifteen years of dust accumulation from her ironing board. Now we can't promise that you will enjoy ironing, but you should see this increase in daily stamina. All other forms of dieting tend to leave you with low energy reserves.

More Lab Results

At the end of the fourth week, our volunteers returned for another battery of fasting blood tests. They did this every four weeks until the end of the twelve–week study. The participants were all anxious to see their cholesterol results. After all, they had always been told to cut their fat intake and we were forcing a high-fat diet on them. The results were remarkable. In general, there was a more than 50 percent reduction in their fasting triglyceride levels even at four weeks into the diet. This showed that the conversion of their metabolism from a carbohydrate-burning to a fat-burning machine really worked. People who have problems with their serum triglyceride levels are classified as having type IV or type IIb lipoproteinemia (having abnormal levels of lipoproteins in the blood). We have known for decades that this is a carbohydrate-induced condition. That message seems to have gotten lost with the high-carbohydrate, low-fat diet craze of the 1990s. Our volunteers, although they had normal triglyceride levels at the beginning of the study, nevertheless demonstrated that most of the triglycerides in the blood have nothing to do with dietary fat intake. Rather, they are the product of carbohydrate metabolism.

How about our one volunteer with the initial triglyceride level of more than 800 mg/dL? At four weeks into the diet, this participant had a fasting triglyceride level of 170 mg/dL. That response is just what a doctor would like to see, and it was a response seen without drugs, with diet alone.

There was little change in the LDL (low-density lipoprotein) and HDL (high-density lipoprotein) cholesterol levels at four weeks. Thus, the high-fat and high dietary cholesterol intake (at least by today's standards) did not cause the participants any harm in terms of blood lipids. However, there was improvement in the volunteers who started with elevated levels of liver enzymes. By the end of the twelve-week study, every participant had normal liver enzyme results. All other tests did not change significantly and confirmed that nutritional markers did not worsen in any way on this diet.

As the diet progressed week after week, the story did not change with regard to the way the subjects felt about the diet.

Finally, at the end of the twelve weeks, we found significant reduction in the total cholesterol and triglyceride levels with a small reduction in the levels of LDL cholesterol, the type of cholesterol that is associated with cardiac risk. The HDL (or "good" cholesterol) levels remained, on average, unchanged. So the diet tended to reduce the cardiac risk associated with total and LDL cholesterol levels.

However, at that point, the diet by itself did not raise protective HDL cholesterol levels; nor did it lower HDL levels. We have looked into this issue of modifying LDL cholesterol and raising HDL cholesterol levels and believe that increasing levels of fiber, garlic, and vitamin E in the diet, as well as increased exercise, may help.

What about Weight Loss?

Yes, our volunteers did lose weight (otherwise there would be no purpose for this book). The range of weight loss for the twenty-four people who completed the twelve-week study was from a low of four pounds to a high of forty-five pounds. The average weight loss at twelve weeks was around twenty pounds, which was about a 10 percent reduction in body weight for this group. Not bad for a diet without much hardship.

Remember, by comparison, a recent dietary "miracle" drug you may have seen advertised on TV, which promises weight losses of less than 10 percent after one year of use. And it has side effects of bloating, diarrhea, and fecal incontinence.

The weight loss was not linear. No one lost two pounds per week, every week. Some weeks there was no weight loss, and other weeks there was remarkable weight loss. Those little plateaus were discouraging to the volunteers, but analysis of their food intake could usually provide a reason. One cheated at her son's birthday party. Another cheated at a beer and pizza party. Other plateaus had less obvious causes. One woman had severe arthritis, and her physician prescribed nonsteroidal anti-inflammatory drugs. That was the end of the rapid weight loss for that woman. Several of the postmenopausal women who were taking hormone-replacement therapy had the slowest weight loss. They still lost weight, and they still had all the positive feelings while on the diet. Their loss was just slower. Men lost the same average weight as women.

There was no predictor that could forecast who would lose the most weight. Not even calorie intake affected the results. The person who lost the most weight ate an average of 1,200 calories per day, but the runner-up ate 2,600 calories per day. They were all individuals who responded to the diet in their own way and lost weight at their own rate. Importantly, all weight loss came from fat stores. Because we measured each volunteer's waist and hip dimensions at the beginning and end of the study, we were able to see an average of five inches lost in the waist, precisely where you would expect to find fat loss.

An exit poll conducted at the end of the study showed no negative comments. Everyone felt better. Everyone lost some weight. Everyone lost inches in the waist. And they all knew how they could solve their own weight problem successfully.

What were the beneficial effects most cited apart from the weight loss?

They had no more bloating after a meal.
They had no need for antacids; digestion improved.
They had abundant energy.
Food no longer played a central role in their lives.
They had fewer vague aches and pains.

This diet was well received and easy to comply with. The high monounsaturated fat levels did indeed protect all the participants from rising cholesterol levels, and the low carbohydrate levels of the diet alleviated many of the problems of hyperinsulinemia and insulin resistance.

From additional observations and personal experience over the longer haul, we found that we could make additional changes, such as lowering the LDL cholesterol with garlic and increasing fiber levels and raising the HDL cholesterol levels with vitamin E naturally or with supplements. Although these issues were not deliberately stressed in the original diet plan, they may offer additional benefits of dietary modification.

STUDY WITH PEOPLE WITH TYPE 2 DIABETES

AS DESCRIBED IN the previous section, we had shown that our diet was safe and successful in nondiabetic obese volunteers. We also wanted to see if it would be safe and successful in people with type 2 diabetes. So in 2002 we conducted a small pilot study of patients with this disease, comparing our results with the results obtained when the same patients followed the American Diabetes Association (ADA) diet.

We recruited six volunteers who were obese and had type 2 diabetes but had not been treated with drugs or insulin. Each volunteer was first placed on the recommended ADA 1,500-calorie diet for six weeks. During this time, each volunteer was given weekly counseling by a registered dietitian. The volunteers also kept diet diaries.

The volunteers were then taught about the Four Corners Diet (then called the GO-Diet) and followed this diet for six weeks, again with weekly counseling by the dietitian.

Blood was obtained before the study and at three-week intervals throughout the study; twenty-four-hour urine samples were collected before the diet therapy and at six-week intervals. Although only four of the six subjects completed the study, results demonstrated that the diet had no deleterious effect.

Fasting blood glucose levels and serum fructosamine levels (a blood test to measure short-term blood glucose control) were lower on the Four Corners Diet than on the ADA diet, indicating better glycemic control on the Four Corners Diet. Both diets promoted weight loss.

On the Four Corners Diet, tests of creatinine clearance demonstrated no harm to kidney function, and in every case the diet lowered the excretion of albumin into the urine (excreting albumin into urine is a sign of kidney damage). Blood studies showed no deterioration in any parameters measured and showed great improvement in serum fasting triglyceride levels.

We conclude from this pilot study that the Four Corners Diet may be a safe alternative to the standard ADA diet for people with type 2 diabetes who are controlling their disease by diet.

The number of volunteers in this pilot study was low, and the time period was relatively short, so large-scale studies are needed to demonstrate the efficacy of the Four Corners Diet in helping people with type 2 diabetes achieve the goal of long-term glycemic control. The short-term results do suggest that it will.

THIRTEEN

Science: The Details

IN EARLIER CHAPTERS, we outlined some of the topics covered here. For some of you, those brief summaries will be enough. But for those interested in a more in-depth understanding of various aspects of the diet, here are some more details.

METABOLIC SYNDROME

SOME PEOPLE ARE just overweight and otherwise healthy, but many overweight people exhibit a constellation of symptoms that has been named metabolic syndrome or insulin resistance syndrome, also called syndrome X or metabolic syndrome X.

Different organizations define this syndrome slightly differently. A recent definition, published in 2003 by a task force from both the American Association of Clinical Endocrinologists and the American College of Endocrinology, defines the syndrome as including impaired glucose tolerance, insulin resistance, and two or more from the following four other components:

- ❖ Hypertension (blood pressure equal to or greater than 160/90)
- ❖ Microalbuminuria
- ❖ Central obesity (waist/hip ratio greater than 0.9 for males or 0.85 for females, with a BMI greater than 30)
- ❖ Dyslipidemia (triglycerides greater than 150 mg/dL and/or HDL cholesterol less than 39 for females or 35 for males)

Many other surrogate markers have been proposed, including elevated uric acid, abnormalities in clotting factors, markers of inflammation such as C-reactive protein (as measured with a high-sensitivity test), and a liver enzyme called gamma-glutamyl transpeptidase.

The cause or causes of the metabolic syndrome are unknown. But whatever the causes, this diet should relieve most of the symptoms.

LAB TESTS AND LIPID SYNDROMES

WE SUGGESTED IN Chapter 4 that you ask your physician for a full lipid profile and tests for glucose and creatinine levels. You will usually be asked to give blood when you're fasting, meaning you haven't had anything to eat for about eight to twelve hours. You should not drink any alcohol at least twenty-four hours prior to the test. The low-density lipoprotein (LDL) and high-density lipoprotein (HDL) cholesterol levels are not affected much by the nonfasting state, but the triglycerides are very dependent on the time since your last meal. Hence a fasting test is recommended. If you do give blood in a nonfasting state, your glucose levels as well as your triglyceride levels (and insulin levels if your doctors want to measure those) may be very different from the results you'd get if you were fasting.

What lipid results do we look for? The National Cholesterol Education Program (2002) has recommended the following guidelines for fasting lipid levels:

- ❖ Total cholesterol should be less than 200 mg/dL.

❖ HDL cholesterol should be greater than 39 mg/dL in men and women. If the HDL cholesterol level is more than 60 mg/dL, it is felt to be protective against cardiac disease, that is, a *negative* risk factor.
❖ Triglycerides should be less than 150 mg/dL.
❖ LDL cholesterol should be less than 130 mg/dL. If you have a history of angina, known coronary artery disease, or diabetes, or have had a heart attack, the LDL should be less than 100 mg/dL.

If your LDL level is high without an elevation of the triglyceride levels, this diet may or may not reduce your cholesterol levels even though it reduces your weight. Adding garlic and more fiber to the diet may help, but if, after a two- to three-month trial of the diet, a repeat analysis of the serum lipids does not show improvement, you should ask your doctor about cholesterol-lowering drugs. This diet will not make the LDL levels worse, but just reducing your weight may not be enough to reduce this cardiac risk factor in your situation.

If your triglycerides are high and your HDL cholesterol is below 40 mg/dL, you will greatly benefit from this diet. You probably have metabolic syndrome. If your triglycerides are high and your HDL level is normal, you may have Fredrickson's type IV lipoproteinemia. Both of these syndromes are very carbohydrate-sensitive, and this diet should normalize your serum lipids.

If your report mentions that your serum was milky and your triglyceride level was in the thousands, you should seek medical intervention. This condition can be due to a variety of causes including alcoholism, obesity, diabetes mellitus, uremia, nephrotic syndrome, pancreatitis, glycogen storage diseases, or drugs such as steroids. The diet may help you, but it should be followed under strict medical supervision to prevent any undesirable side effects. The exact biochemical defect that causes this condition is unknown. It may be due to a reduction in levels of the enzymes that break down fats in the blood (lipoprotein lipases) or to defective mechanisms of removal of the lipoprotein particles, or both.

How about the glucose levels? According to current standards, if your fasting blood glucose level is below 126 mg/dL, you're not diabetic. However, most healthy people do not have fasting levels that high. Normal fasting blood glucose levels are now considered to be up to 99. Anyone with a fasting level of 100 or more can be considered to have prediabetes. If you have prediabetes, you are at high risk of becoming diabetic.

Postprandial (nonfasting) blood glucose levels are considered diabetic if they're greater than 200 mg/dL on a random blood glucose test, or if they don't fall below 140 mg/dL by two hours during a glucose tolerance test (see Chapter 12).

Fasting and postprandial insulin levels have not proved to be useful in diagnosis of either insulin resistance or diabetes, so we no longer recommend insulin testing.

WHY THIS DIET IS LOW CARBOHYDRATE: THE ROLE OF INSULIN

VERY LOW-CALORIE and low-fat diets fail long term in obese subjects almost 100 percent of the time. Yes, the dieters initially lose weight, but within a year or so, most of them regain the weight and end up heavier than when they started. They were doomed to failure even before they began. What drives their bodies back up the scale?

You remember that otherwise healthy overweight people in general suffer from hyperinsulinemia, meaning too much insulin in the blood. The scientific literature is crammed full of research papers describing this situation. There is nothing new about it. So why has it been ignored by mainstream medical practice? It is probably because the problem of weight was not epidemic in our society until recently. In that same time frame, we have become preoccupied with a bystander called cholesterol that just happened to be in the wrong place at the wrong time. Over the past twenty-five years, we have been barraged with propaganda imploring, cajoling, and threatening us to cut out fats and red meat from our diet and eat more carbohydrates, especially so-called complex carbohydrates.

The message was simple, and food processors and agribusiness benefited. Low-fat foods are usually high-carbohydrate foods. Those carbohydrates are often sugars and starches, both of which quickly raise blood sugar levels. The carbohydrates in processed foods are much cheaper than proteins. They also tend to be almost addictive. Maybe they're not exactly like heroin or nicotine, but if you eat the fast-acting carbohydrates in processed foods, you produce a lot of insulin, which causes your blood sugar level to fall, which makes you very hungry, so you eat more carbohydrates. Inadvertently, a vicious circle is set up.

This cycle of sugar–insulin–more sugar–more insulin starts off pretty innocently. Most people can handle it. They have the genetic makeup to adapt to this type of diet. But a substantial minority, those with a genetic tendency to insulin resistance, can take it for only so long.

When the muscle cells are insulin resistant and don't take up enough glucose from the blood, the levels of glucose in the blood rise too high. This makes the pancreas, which produces the insulin, produce even more insulin than normal to try to overcome the insulin resistance. More insulin tells the body to store more fat. Increased fat in the body causes more insulin resistance. This makes the pancreas produce even more insulin resistance. You get the picture. You're caught in a vicious cycle that leads to ever-increasing hyperinsulinemia.

If you have the appropriate genes and you get into this cycle, there is only one outcome: type 2 diabetes. Over 80 percent of people with type 2 diabetes are overweight, and a substantial proportion of overweight people (probably more than 50 percent) will become diabetic. We are embarking on an outbreak of diabetes that will reach epidemic proportions.

Some people become hyperinsulinemic early in life. Babies born to mothers with uncontrolled diabetes are hyperinsulinemic. Because of this, they are often extremely large when born, and they also become heavy later in life. Other people become hyperinsulinemic at the onset of puberty, become fat adolescents, thin out for early adulthood, and then later go into their middle-aged spread.

What is happening? What does control of blood sugar have to do with your being fat?

To answer this question, we must get a little technical. First, think of hormones as e-mail and receptors (structures on cells that bind hormones and transmit their signals to the cells) as e-mail addresses. Insulin is a hormone (e-mail) produced by the pancreas. Most people have heard about insulin in relation to diabetes, in which insulin is either deficient (type 1 diabetes, in which people must take insulin injections) or ineffective because of insulin resistance (type 2 diabetes, in which insulin resistance is usually the major problem). Insulin's main claim to fame is controlling blood sugar levels.

But that isn't the only effect of insulin. Many tissues have insulin receptors (e-mail addresses that will accept the e-mail), and the function of insulin varies with the tissue. In muscle cells, the insulin is mainly concerned with causing the cells to take glucose out of the bloodstream and put it into storage as a molecule called glycogen. Glycogen is animal starch. It is a huge molecule made by linking many glucose molecules together.

In the liver, glycogen is used to store excess energy until it is needed by other cells in the body. The glycogen in the liver can tide you over between meals. After a meal, increased glucose levels in the blood stimulate the pancreas to release insulin. In the liver, the insulin stimulates the liver cells to make a lot of glycogen; at the same time it inhibits the breakdown of existing glycogen into glucose. Then several hours after the meal, as the blood sugar levels fall, the pancreas stops producing a lot of insulin and starts producing another hormone, glucagon. Glucagon does the opposite of insulin: it tells the liver to stop storing glycogen and to break it down into glucose. The liver releases this glucose into the bloodstream in sufficient quantities to maintain your blood sugar level within normal limits.

In a healthy person, a complex system of feedback loops using these e-mail messages (hormones) and e-mail addresses (hormone receptors) keeps the blood glucose level within a very narrow range.

When you have insulin resistance (hyperinsulinemia), different organs may have different degrees of insulin resistance. For example, the insulin receptors on your liver cells may not be as resistant as those on muscle cells. The insulin resistance in the muscle cells means they can't take up as much glucose as they normally would, and that means your pancreas will produce insulin as fast as its little enzyme factory can work to try to overcome the resistance. You've become hyperinsulinemic.

But if your liver cells aren't quite as insulin resistant as the muscle cells, all that extra insulin will give them a superstrong message to MAKE GLYCOGEN. You may even be able to sense this situation. If you are hyperinsulinemic and eat a big pasta meal with plenty of garlic bread, followed by pie or ice cream, you are going to suffer. The better it tasted going down, the more you will get that bloated feeling about one to two hours later. Your liver is just stuffing those sugar molecules into glycogen until the cells begin to swell. Some of the excess sugar is then converted into fat, which is temporarily stored in the liver. Your liver gets so big you think you are going to burst. The process is relentless. Your liver gets so stuffed that after a high-carbohydrate meal you can see the skin across your stomach becoming taut and shiny while you have difficulty breathing. Now that's bloating. Sound familiar?

While the liver is producing its glycogen, it is also converting some excess sugar into fat, which is exported into the bloodstream and carried to the fat cells for storage. The fat cells may also be less insulin resistant than the muscle cells, so they will also come under the influence of those high insulin levels, which urge them to remove the fat as well as glucose from the blood and store everything as body fat.

TWO ANTAGONISTS

We've mentioned that high insulin levels in the blood (hyperinsulinemia) can cause problems with your health. Carbohydrates make insulin levels go up.

However, because insulin is also needed to process amino acids, the building blocks of proteins, proteins also make insulin levels go up, and some critics of low carbohydrate levels claim that eating a lot of protein will cause just as much damage from high insulin levels as eating a lot of carbohydrate foods.

But insulin levels alone do not govern its actions. Insulin has an antagonist, called glucagon, that in general does just exactly the opposite of what insulin does. Insulin says "Store fat," and glucagon says, "Don't store fat." Insulin says, "Don't break down the fat you've already got stored," and glucagon says, "Break that fat down." Insulin tells the liver to take glucose out of the bloodstream and store it. Glucagon tells the liver to make glucose and send it into the bloodstream.

And in general, *it's the ratio of insulin to glucagon that determines what the effect of these hormone levels will be.*

Now, when you eat carbohydrates, your body produces more insulin. When you eat protein, your body also produces more insulin. But when you eat protein, your body also produces more glucagon. So the net effect of protein on blood sugar levels in anyone who does not have diabetes (and hence can't produce enough insulin) is negligible.

Thus the higher levels of insulin caused by eating carbohydrates have different effects than the higher levels of insulin caused by eating protein, which also causes levels of the counterbalancing glucagon to rise.

Sometimes fat remains in the liver and can cause a condition known as steatohepatitis, which is a mild inflammation of the liver caused by fat. If you are obese and have slightly elevated liver enzymes (ALT and AST), this may be an indication that you are developing steatohepatitis.

Protein packets called lipoproteins carry the fat that is made in the liver into the bloodstream. We've mentioned some of these lipoproteins before: high-density lipoprotein (HDL, the "good" cholesterol) and low-density lipoprotein (LDL, the "bad" cholesterol). The one that carries the fat away from the liver is called very low density lipoprotein, or VLDL. The VLDL travels through the bloodstream until it reaches tissues that want to burn that fat for energy.

Fat consists of long molecules called fatty acids hooked onto a small molecule called glycerin. Fat can't get through cell membranes; it's too big. So the tissues that want to get fat from the lipoproteins have to use enzymes called lipases to break the fats down into glycerin and fatty acids, which can get across cell membranes. Once in the cell, the fatty acids may be reassembled into fat.

These important lipases are present in arterial and capillary walls, anchored by complex carbohydrates called glycosaminoglycans. Once the lipases have removed the fat from the VLDL particles, the remnant VLDL particles can then go through a series of interactions with other lipoproteins in the plasma. After taking on a load of cholesterol, they become LDL. It is these cholesterol-rich LDL particles, especially those damaged by free radicals, that can be deposited in the arterial walls, leading to atherosclerosis.

In people with diabetes, and probably also those who are obese (as we have already discussed, obesity and diabetes are kissing cousins), the VLDL remnant particle itself may be deposited in the artery wall. This is probably one reason most people with type 2 diabetes die from coronary artery disease.

You remember that the liver stores glycogen to use to make glucose when blood glucose levels fall too low. When you don't eat for a long time and most of the liver's glycogen is used up, the fat cells start converting some of their fat into fatty acids, which they release into the bloodstream to be sent to various tissues to be burned for energy.

Thus, through a complex system of checks and balances, in a healthy person all the cells of the body can receive just enough energy—either glucose or fatty acids—to satisfy their energy needs.

However, if you have hyperinsulinemia, the process of blood glucose control tends to overshoot the mark. After a meal, your blood sugar level falls too far or too fast, perhaps because insulin's balancing hormone, glucagon—which in a healthy person tells the liver to break down glycogen and release glucose into the bloodstream to keep blood glucose levels from going too low—can't work properly in the presence of all this insulin. This can cause symptoms of hypoglycemia (low blood sugar)—shakiness, sweating, rapid heartbeat, anxiety, and a feeling of nervousness or impending doom. But in most cases it simply makes you look for food. Usually you're not seeking carrots or celery sticks. You crave the quickly absorbed carbohydrates that will raise your blood sugar level fast: a couple of cookies, a bag of pretzels, a slice of cake or pie. Experience has taught you that these are the foods that make you feel better when your blood sugar levels go too low.

Now you should see why your eating problem is driven by insulin, why the low-fat, high-carbohydrate diets don't work for you. Unless you address your insulin problem, your weight is going to stay with you. There is nothing else it can do. The problem is not your willpower; it's nature, and you can't fight Mother Nature. Because you have insulin resistance, you need to keep your net carbohydrate intake below the threshold that will stimulate increasingly higher insulin release.

WHY THIS DIET EMPHASIZES HIGH MONOUNSATURATED FATS

BY NOW, EVERYONE has probably heard of the association between fats containing saturated fatty acids and heart disease, cancer, and possibly diabetes. But as noted in Chapter 3, all the studies were based on diets that were high in saturated fat but also relatively high in carbohydrates. We have not found any study showing deleterious effects of saturated fats on people who eat a diet low in carbohydrates, but we are taking a conservative view and recommend a limit on saturated fat.

When you consume a diet high in carbohydrate, your plasma cholesterol level is much more dependent on your fat consumption than on your cholesterol intake. But when you eat a very low-carbohydrate diet, most people (about 70 percent) find that their plasma cholesterol levels are dramatically reduced even when they eat a lot of fat.

Numerous books and papers have been published describing the effects of the hunter-gatherer type of diet. Tribal peoples who eat only meat, fish, and the few seasonal vegetables, nuts, and fruits available in their habitat tend to have low incidences of heart disease and diabetes. The point of these tribal diets is that although some can be high in fat, they are simultaneously low in carbohydrates.

One author of a popular low-carbohydrate diet book does warn that about 30 percent of people are fat-sensitive and their cholesterol levels will go up if they follow his diet, which doesn't limit saturated fat. However, we have found in the literature and shown in our studies that a high consumption of monounsaturated fats can counteract this effect. There are numerous publications to justify this claim.

OMEGA-3 AND OMEGA-6 OILS

We've talked a lot about saturated fat and monounsaturated fat in this book. The other kind of fat is polyunsaturated fat. Polyunsaturated fat comes in two major classes, called omega-3 and omega-6. You need to have a certain amount of both these polyunsaturated fats in your diet because your body can't make them.

Good sources of polyunsaturated fats are fresh vegetables, nuts, vegetable oils, and seafood.

In nonindustrialized diets, the ratio of omega-6 to omega-3 fats is about 2:1. Some people think Americans are eating too many omega-6 fats and not enough of the omega-3. Hence the more you can increase your consumption of omega-3–rich foods, the better.

Good omega-3 sources are cold-water fish and a few vegetable foods including flaxseed, walnuts, and purslane, a "weed" that is grown as a vegetable in other parts of the world.

We've used the word *fat* here for the various unsaturated vegetable oils. Technically, a fat is solid at room temperature and an oil is liquid. As a general rule, the more unsaturated a fat is, the more liquid it is at room temperature.

Because "room temperature" at the equator is warmer than "room temperature" in the Arctic, cold-water fish tend to have highly unsaturated fats. If they didn't, they'd be so solid they couldn't swim. And tropical plants such as coconut tend to have highly saturated fats. If they didn't, they'd melt in the sun.

There is evidence of a relationship between the composition of dietary fatty acids and serum insulin levels. Researchers measured plasma phospholipid fatty acid levels, an indicator of the fatty acid composition of the diet, in 4,304 middle-aged nondiabetic adults. They found that fasting insulin levels, a marker of insulin resistance (although not sufficiently accurate to be used in clinical diagnosis), were strongly and positively associated with the saturated fatty acid percentage in plasma phospholipids; moderately and inversely associated with the monounsaturated percentage; and not appreciably associated with the polyunsaturated fat percentage.

These data are consistent with studies showing that the fatty acid composition of cell membranes modulates insulin action. They support the hypothesis that increased habitual saturated fat intake is a risk factor for hyperinsulinemia. It should follow that monounsaturated fats would relieve this problem.

Monounsaturated fats also seem to provide a degree of protection against some cancers. One of the conclusions of a case-controlled study was that unsaturated fatty acids protect against breast cancer, possibly because intake of these nutrients is also closely correlated to a high intake of vegetables. The findings also suggested a possible increased risk of breast cancer in southern European populations whose diet is largely based on starch (carbohydrates).

WHY DIETARY FIBER IS IMPORTANT

AS EXPLAINED EARLIER, fiber consists of very complex carbohydrates, both soluble and insoluble, that humans are unable to digest. However, bacteria that can digest this fiber live in your colon, as well as in the rumen of ruminant herbivorous animals such as sheep and cows, and even in the intestines of termites. In ruminants and termites, the bacteria digest the fiber, especially cellulose, and produce fatty acids that the termites and ruminants can use.

In humans, most of the fiber passes right through the digestive tract. But, as described in Chapter 3, fiber can help with constipation. It can also help reduce cholesterol levels. Bile is made from cholesterol derivatives called bile acids. The bile is secreted into the intestine, where it helps solubilize fatty foods. But farther down the intestine, much of the bile is reabsorbed and the bile acids are recycled. Dietary fiber binds the bile acids, preventing reabsorption, so the liver uses more cholesterol to make more bile acids. The result is lower levels of cholesterol in the blood.

Studies have also implied that fiber has a protective effect against many cancers. Experimental and epidemiological evidence suggests that increased dietary fiber is associated with decreased breast cancer risk, but little is known about the role played by different types of fiber, and particularly mixtures of soluble and insoluble fibers similar to those consumed by human populations, in reducing breast cancer risk. High intake of fiber may suppress bacterial breakdown of biliary estrogen conjugates to free (absorbable) estrogens in the colon and thus may decrease the availability of circulating estrogens necessary for the development and growth of breast cancers.

THE TWO FACES OF FIBER

As we've emphasized in this book, fibers are wonderful additions to your diet. However, there are a few caveats you should be aware of.

Insoluble fibers like wheat bran contain compounds called phytates that can bind minerals like calcium. They could also bind certain drugs. What this means is that you should not eat a meal with a lot of bran at the same time you're taking calcium supplements or other medications. If you take the pills a couple of hours before or after the bran, you shouldn't have a problem.

If you have the diabetic complication called gastroparesis, meaning that your stomach doesn't empty as fast as it should, a high-fiber diet is not a good choice for you. On the other hand, if you don't have gastroparesis, a high-fiber diet may help you control your blood glucose levels so you never develop this complication.

A study on rats looked at this effect. The study evaluated the effect of wheat bran (an insoluble fiber) and psyllium (a soluble fiber) alone and in combination on overall estrogen status and on the induction of mammary tumors in rats treated with a cancer-causing agent. The results demonstrated that as the level of psyllium relative to that of wheat bran increased, the total tumor number and multiplicity of mammary tumors in rats decreased. The authors concluded that the addition of a 4 percent: 4 percent mixture of an insoluble (wheat bran) fiber and a soluble (psyllium) fiber to a high-fat diet provided the maximal tumor-inhibiting effects in this breast tumor model. Although increasing levels of dietary psyllium were associated with decreased bacterial enzyme activity, these changes were not reflected in decreased circulating levels of tumor-promoting estrogens. Therefore, the mechanism or mechanisms by which mixtures of soluble and insoluble dietary fibers protect against mammary tumorigenesis still remains to be clarified.

The tumor-fighting potential of high-fiber, low-digestible-carbohydrate foods such as flaxseeds makes these foods an ideal component of the Four Corners Diet.

WHY KEFIR, YOGURT, AND OTHER FERMENTED MILK PRODUCTS ARE IMPORTANT

LACTOBACILLUS AND SIMILAR organisms are the bacteria that convert milk to products like buttermilk, cheese, yogurt, and kefir. As mentioned in Chapter 3, a steady source of live *Lactobacillus* organisms in the diet will help maintain a healthy bowel and help prevent overgrowth of the bowel and the vagina by such organisms as *Candida albicans*, a notorious yeast whose presence can give many vague symptoms. The bacteria may have additional benefits as well.

The milk-fermenting organisms have recently been found to stimulate the immune system, and keeping the immune system functioning properly is probably key to the body's natural defenses against infectious diseases and cancer. This research has shown that among its many good qualities, these bacteria also stimulate the body to produce important immune-response chemicals called cytokines. These "might promote a continuous state of alertness against attack by viruses and other pathogenic organisms," according to the authors of one study.

Note that yogurt and kefir cultures may contain several different types of bacteria. The types that are added to all yogurts to ferment the milk are *Lactobacillus bulgaricus* and *Streptococcus thermophilus*. *Lactobacillus lactis* is added to milk to produce cottage cheese. However, many of these bacteria don't survive the acidic conditions of the stomach. Hence some manufacturers have begun to add additional types of bacteria to their yogurt, including *Lactobacillus acidophilus*, *Lactobacillus casei*,

Lactobacillus reuteri, and *Bifidobacterium bifidum*. These are considered to be probiotic bacteria, as they can survive the harsh conditions of the stomach. Kefir contains additional probiotic organisms, including beneficial yeasts.

To get the maximum benefit from cultured milk products, it's important that you choose a reliable manufacturer. You should also make sure the product says it contains live cultures. If possible, buy a product that contains some of the extra types of probiotic bacteria.

KETONES

MANY PEOPLE REPORT an increased feeling of well-being on the Four Corners Diet. Why? This is a difficult question to answer with facts, but it may have to do with the ketogenic state of a low carbohydrate intake. When the body reaches a state of carbohydrate depletion, it starts to burn fat for fuel. This happens when you fast (the ultimate low-carbohydrate diet) or perform long strenuous exercise, or in some abnormal situations such as uncontrolled type 1 diabetes, when there is no available insulin to force the sugars into the cells.

Burning fatty acids for energy is a normal function of cells. It occurs in little power factories within the cells called mitochondria. The fatty acids, which contain long chains of carbon atoms, are chopped up two carbon atoms at a time in a process call beta-oxidation. For example, an eighteen-carbon chain fatty acid will be broken down into nine two-carbon pieces. These two-carbon pieces then get attached to a molecule called coenzyme A to produce acetyl-coenzyme A (acetyl-CoA for short). Acetyl-CoA molecules are the primary building blocks for new fatty acids and cholesterol synthesis.

Under normal feeding conditions, when there are plenty of carbohydrates around, most of the acetyl-CoA gets burned up in the cells' major energy-producing cycle called the tricarboxylic acid or citric acid or Krebs cycle. In that case, almost all these two–carbon compounds end up as carbon dioxide, water, and energy. This is the usual way that we derive energy from carbohydrates, fats, and proteins. Indeed, many fad supplements, such as isocitric acid, which claim to aid in weight reduction, are components of the citric acid cycle.

In times of carbohydrate starvation, however, when fats are being chopped up for energy, there is an excess of acetyl-CoA molecules, and they get shunted off into an alternative pathway in the mitochondria and end up as compounds called ketone bodies and carbon dioxide. This process is called ketosis.

Two main ketone bodies are produced. One is called acetoacetic acid and the other is named beta-hydroxybutyric acid (HBA). Acetoacetic acid can spontaneously break down to form acetone, and this is the compound that can give people on this diet a faint but distinct acetone smell on their breath.

The cells in your body, including brain cells, can burn ketone bodies for fuel after a short period of adaptation in which they learn to make the enzymes needed to process the ketone bodies. If you're eating a lot of fat, however, you're producing more ketone bodies than your cells can use, and some of them get excreted in the urine.

The ketones in the urine can be detected with special dipsticks (Ketostix). Some other low-carbohydrate diets advocate using ketone test strips to detect these ketones in the urine as a sign that you are really burning fats. However, these sticks, which are expensive, detect only the acetoacetic acid and acetone, which constitute less than 20 percent of the ketones produced. The HBA goes totally undetected by this test. Many people never produce enough acetoacetic acid to cause these sticks to turn color, yet testing their blood for HBA shows plenty of ketones.

We therefore suggest that you don't bother with ketone test strips. They may be interesting for you to use as a check for ketosis, but ketosis has nothing to do with your rate of weight loss. We have seen people positive for urine ketones not losing weight, and people who are negative for ketones rapidly losing weight. Save your money.

One final word about ketones. Some people will tell you that producing ketones is dangerous. This is just misinformation. They are confusing ketosis (ketones in the blood) with ketoacidosis (extremely high levels of ketones in the blood along with an acidic condition), which occurs in people with uncontrolled diabetes. This diet does *not* produce ketoacidosis. Unless you have uncontrolled diabetes, your body's fail-safe mechanisms will stop the production of ketones before they reach dangerous, acid-producing levels.

Ketones may have two bad side effects. The first is the ketone headache. When you begin a ketogenic (ketosis-producing) diet, or when you fast without food or water, the ketones can build up to a level that can affect the brain. The brain can use ketones as fuel, but it normally doesn't get many ketones, so it takes a few days for it to adapt.

Think of it like a factory that makes apple juice. The equipment for squeezing and filtering the fruit is geared to handling apples. Suppose there were no more apples, but a convoy of trucks came by carrying grapes. It shouldn't take long to convert that factory to efficiently handle the grapes to make grape juice, but it would take a short period of adjustment to tool up for the special processes that efficient grape squeezing would need.

It's the same with the brain. It can handle ketones, but it takes a day or two for the machinery to gear up to handle the load. During that time you may get the ketone headache. It goes away all by itself. Drinking plenty of liquids helps, and if all else fails, an over-the-counter headache pill will work. Even when fully on the diet, if you don't drink enough water, you can get an occasional ketone headache. Indeed, that is one of the self-tests for adequate fluid intake.

The other side effect is acetone breath. Again, drinking enough fluid should dilute this effect. How much fluid intake is adequate? Probably no fewer than six to eight glasses of water per day. This can consist of water, pop, tea, coffee, and other drinks. However, be aware that caffeine is a diuretic and will cause the kidneys to get rid of fluids. Try to drink decaffeinated or caffeine-free beverages most of the time. However, if you must have your morning java, it's okay. If you drink a lot of coffee, drink extra water to compensate.

The ketones have one or two very pleasant side effects. They give you a sense of well-being and they suppress your appetite. So the fewer carbohydrates you eat, the higher the level of your ketosis and the less you will want to eat.

One high-carbohydrate meal will remove all the ketones from your body very rapidly. It can take a day or two to get back to where you were. Because you won't have the ketones in your blood, you will probably eat more and stop your weight loss, at least temporarily. If you eat two or more consecutive high-carbohydrate meals, the weight will start piling back on, and you will have to return to the first-phase transition diet to get back on track. Even if this happens, don't lose faith in yourself. Sure, you had a moment of weakness, but you did it once and you can get back on track.

MORE SCIENCE

EACH RESEARCH PAPER in the scientific literature contributes a small piece of the puzzle of optimal nutrition, but when combined they present a deafening condemnation of some of the nutritional advice currently advocated by governmental and academic societies. Why have those august bodies not modified their positions? It is not because these papers were published in obscure journals. Indeed, most of them have been published in the most prestigious journals of the medical profession. It is not because the research results are in doubt. Rather, it is probably an inability to admit that the advice so freely administered in the past may in fact be contributing to the epidemics of obesity and type 2 diabetes that we see today. Yes, the "heart-friendly diets" may be fine for a majority of the population, perhaps even a large majority. But what about the misery caused to the 25 to 30 percent of the population it will harm?

What's the proof? Well, let's just skim some of the reports.

In November 1997, the *Journal of the American Medical Association* published a paper that demonstrated that moderate restriction of dietary fat intake achieved meaningful and sustained LDL cholesterol reductions in hypercholesterolemic (HC; high cholesterol levels in the blood) subjects and apolipoprotein B (apolipoprotein B is the lipoprotein associated with LDL, the "bad" cholesterol, and high levels are considered undesirable) reductions in both HC subjects and those with combined hyperlipidemia (CHL; people having both high cholesterol levels and high triglyceride levels). Their conclusions were that "more extreme restriction of fat intake offers little further advantage in HC or CHL subjects and potentially undesirable effects in HC subjects." These authors demonstrated that lowering the fat content below the 30 percent of calories actually caused harm to those in the HC group.

Did they question whether 30 percent fat calories and 50 to 60 percent carbohydrate calories was a diet suitable for hypertriglyceridemic (high triglyceride levels in the blood) subjects even though all those in the CHL group remained hypertriglyceridemic and some of those in the CH group became hypertriglyceridemic while on the diet? No.

A paper in the *American Journal of Clinical Nutrition* demonstrated an increase from 8 to 13 percent in the number of women with an undesirable (that means low) HDL cholesterol level after going on the American Heart Association diet. These authors write that "a decline in the HDL-cholesterol concentration in response to a high-carbohydrate, low-fat diet is potentially harmful for older women who are at a heightened risk for coronary artery disease." They also state that "a low-fat diet without substantial weight loss is not beneficial for improving lipoprotein lipid risk factors in obese, postmenopausal women with normal lipid profiles." These authors had the insight to comment that "weight loss without a low-fat diet may increase HDL cholesterol above pretreatment values while also lowering total cholesterol." Did anyone hear of this study on the nightly news broadcast? Why not?

A second study involving only ten individual subjects published in the same journal confirmed these findings and showed that these "untoward metabolic effects of low-fat, high-carbohydrate diets are directly related to degree of insulin resistance." Therefore, women who are overweight to begin with are most likely to increase their risk factors for heart disease by eating a high-carbohydrate diet.

This phenomenon is not limited to postmenopausal women. A paper published in the journal *Pediatrics* also concluded "not only that obese adolescents have lipid abnormalities (elevated serum LDL-C and triglycerides, and reduced HDL-C levels) but also that these abnormalities correlate with the degree of insulin resistance." Again we see the link between obesity, insulin resistance, and serum lipid abnormalities. Are you beginning to get the picture?

How about studies of younger people? One study clearly demonstrated that insulin resistance and hyperinsulinemia coexist in adolescent children with moderate to severe obesity. There are papers that go all the way back to the effects of hyperinsulinism of the fetus caused by gestational diabetes. The story is always the same. In a different study, forty-three adult obese subjects who were assigned to a low-calorie diet, either a high-carbohydrate (45 percent) or a low-carbohydrate (15 percent) one. The weight loss was about the same for both groups after six weeks. However, the low-carbohydrate diet group had significantly lower insulin, cholesterol, and triglyceride levels at the end of the test period. These authors concluded that "consumption of the kind of low-fat, high-carbohydrate diet for weight maintenance advocated by the National Cholesterol Education Program seems to minimize the fall in plasma insulin and triacylglycerol concentrations." Again, more proof that the high-fat, low-carbohydrate diets may be better for weight-loss programs.

The study just cited emphasized calorie restriction. But we find that if we keep the carbohydrate levels low, we can increase the fat intake while maintaining the weight loss. Remember that the right kinds of fats are key.

Perhaps one of the most telling, yet underreported, papers was published in the prestigious *Journal of Pediatrics*. These authors studied fruit juice intake in 116 two-year-old and 107 five-year-old children. They demonstrated that two-year-olds who drank more than 12 fluid ounces of fruit juice per day were three times as likely as their peers (47 percent versus 14 percent) to be short. Also, 32 percent of the juice drinkers had a BMI greater than the 90th percentile for BMI, compared with only 9 percent of children who drank less than 12 fluid ounces of juice per day.

Does this mean that drinking excess fruit juices caused these children to be short and fat? This was not proved by this study. It does bring up the interesting observation that your body's natural satiety (feeling of satisfaction) from real fruit is bypassed when you drink fruit juice. You probably would not eat more than one orange or apple at a time if you were eating the whole fruit, right? But you think nothing of consuming the juice from three, four, or maybe even five oranges or apples when you drink a tall glass of juice. You drink all the carbohydrates and get almost none of the fiber!

Those of you who are old enough may remember that before the 1960s, apples and oranges were tart. Slowly but surely, agribusiness has bred out the tartness and left or increased the sweetness of all fruit. After all, you can sell many more sweet oranges than tart oranges. They have bypassed our natural ability to say, "No more! I am satisfied." You older guys can also remember that fruit used to be only seasonally available. Oranges were available for only a few months. Strawberries were the treat of early summer. And bananas were imported only during short growing seasons. Now, with the improvement of transportation systems, refrigeration, and multinational agribusiness, you can get almost any fruit or vegetable all year round. When you walk into your supermarket, it is perpetual summer. Never in the history of humankind has this happened, and the result is seen on your hips and waist. You can now feed your hyperinsulinism with so-called nutritious fruits and their juices all year round.

Another study in adolescents was published in the journal *Pediatrics*. It demonstrated rapid weight loss in adolescents with little loss in lean body weight when the adolescents were put on a high-protein (80 to 100 grams), low-fat (25 grams), very low-carbohydrate (25 grams) ketogenic diet. This study clearly demonstrated the safety of very low-carbohydrate diets, even in children twelve to fifteen years old.

So why would anyone feed a high-carbohydrate diet to anyone with hyperinsulinemia? Is the defect reversible by continually stimulating the pancreas to produce more insulin? Why do scientists and clinicians continually confuse the well-documented bad effects of a high-fat and high-carbohydrate diet with the clearly demonstrated benefits of a very low-carbohydrate diet?

Everyone should agree that the first priority in treating obesity is normalizing weight. Low-carbohydrate diets do this effectively and quickly, and if you follow the Four Corners Diet, you should do this without increasing any of your lipid risk factors.

What to do in the long term may be debated for years to come. We have no prospective scientific data on the long-term effects of a very low-carbohydrate diet except for anecdotal reports. In fact, we have no long-term studies of any diet at all, except natural studies of populations who have been following one diet or another for generations.

It is logical that if you lose weight on a low-carb diet but then return to the high-carbohydrate diet you were on when you gained all that weight, the latter will produce the same effect that it did originally. So we suggest that eating low carbohydrates—with the appropriate modifications of high monounsaturated fats, high fiber, natural sources of vitamins, minerals, antioxidants, and phytochemicals through several servings of assorted vegetables each day, and fermented milk products—will have to be a permanent dietary change. But can you even think that your former eating habits gave you as much nutrition?

We would like to monitor the long-term benefits of this diet to see if nutrition can promote health over a lifetime. But this may be difficult. After all, would you really want to join such a study if it meant you would have to return to your old way of eating and risk regaining all the weight you'd lost, along with its associated health risks? The best studies are called crossover studies, meaning that the same subjects are given the experimental treatment for a period of time and the control treatment for a period of time. They "cross over" from one to the other. It would be difficult to get volunteers to agree to do a crossover study of the Four Corners Diet after they'd lost weight on the diet and felt so much healthier.

■

A WORD ABOUT EXERCISE

EXERCISING AS LITTLE as brisk walking (walking fast enough to get your heart rate up) daily may have a positive effect on raising HDL (good) cholesterol. Even though exercise alone will not make you lose much weight, we strongly support exercise by brisk walking, starting with ten minutes a day and working up to twenty to thirty minutes every day. A general program of mobility exercising is also advisable.

One good trick to help you get walking is the step counter. For about $20 you can buy a pedometer that you clip on your belt. It tells you how many steps you've walked that day. The goal for people with diabetes is ten thousand steps a day.

Just keep in mind that you should be doing this exercise for its benefits on the general conditioning of the body and for possible effects on raising HDL cholesterol. You should *not* expect the exercise to contribute a lot to your weight loss. The diet is for weight loss.

During our study (see Chapter 12), we specifically forbade the subjects to start an exercise program concurrent with the diet study. Why? We wanted to look strictly at the effects of the diet on weight loss and bio-chemical markers in the blood. Some diet programs have their partici-pants undergo a complete lifestyle change, including a new diet, increased exercise, stress reduction, and other changes. These are all healthy things to do, but then one shouldn't ascribe any positive changes to the diet alone.

If you are significantly overweight, attempting to increase exercise beyond walking may be harmful. Yes, we said harmful. We feel that any exercise program beyond simple brisk walking should be medically super-vised. We support exercise when and how it is recommended by your doctor. You'll get there, but at the right pace, and safely.

■

ANTIOXIDANTS AND FREE RADICALS

ANTIOXIDANTS ARE COMPOUNDS that scavenge "free radicals," sub-stances that can damage cellular DNA and blood components such as lipoproteins. Cells with damaged DNA may not be able to repair them-selves or prevent making copies of themselves, and these mutations can result in tumors or cellular structural damage. In arteries, the altered lipoproteins may lead to increased atherosclerosis, which can lead to strokes and heart attacks. If the affected arteries are in the retinas of your eyes, free radicals may contribute to age-related macular degeneration. If the affected DNA is damaged in the lungs or colon, then tumors in these areas may result.

One important, preventable cause of cellular damage that can affect many organs is cigarette smoking. Another example is excessive exposure to UV light, associated with skin cancers. However, there are other environmental insults that we may not be able to avoid.

A diet rich in antioxidants may help in reducing the burden of free radicals.

FOURTEEN

Frequently Asked Questions

Alcohol

How much alcohol can I have?

It varies, but for women no more than one five-ounce glass of dry wine or one cocktail or one light beer per day; for men, no more than two five-ounce glasses of dry wine or two cocktails or two light beers per day. Remember to use no-carb or low-carb mixers.

Artificial Sweeteners

Can I use artificial sweeteners?

Yes. All artificial sweeteners are okay in cold foods. You must not cook with aspartame (NutraSweet; Equal). In cooking and baking, substitute saccharin (Sugar Twin, Sweet'n Low), acesulfame-K (Sweet One; Sunette), or sucralose (Splenda). If you wish, you can use stevia, which has been approved by the Food and Drug Administration as a supplement, but not specifically as a sweetener. Only buy plain or artificially sweetened yogurt or kefir, diet sodas, or mixers, or make them yourself. Packets of sweeteners have about 1 gram of carbs each. Most tablets and liquids have zero carbs; check labels to make sure the tablets don't contain carbohydrate fillers. The measure-for-measure sweeteners like bulk Splenda and Equal Spoonful (with which 1 teaspoonful is as sweet as 1 teaspoon of table sugar) contain about 0.5 grams of carbs per teaspoonful.

Brans and Flax

Where can I buy wheat or other brans and flaxseeds?
Most health food stores and specialty sections of large food stores carry them. Grind the flaxseeds in your coffee grinder, or keep a special grinder just for this purpose.

Caffeine

Can I take caffeine drinks?
Yes. But keep it to a minimum. Caffeine is a diuretic and causes water loss. This can lead to headaches.

Calories

Do I have to count calories?
No. Your own body will control your food intake when you don't have hunger pangs caused by rapid blood sugar swings.

Cholesterol

Will eating all that fat increase my cholesterol?
No. In most cases it will reduce your cholesterol levels. If you do see a rise, it may be brought back down with garlic and vitamin E supplements. The emphasis on monounsaturated fats and fiber in this diet is the key feature that prevent cholesterol levels from rising.

Constipation

Will this diet be constipating?

No. After the first few days you should emphasize both soluble and insoluble fiber intake and yogurt or kefir. This will bulk the stool. Also drink at least eight glasses of liquids per day.

Diet Safety

Are there any new studies showing that low-carb diets are safe and effective?

Several recent studies have examined the short-term effects of low-carbohydrate diets and—like our study—found no deleterious effects. See References for details.

The important points to remember are that any low-carb diet plan you choose to follow should still be controlled in the amount of saturated fat taken daily and analyzed to ensure that essential nutrients are not neglected. Lowering the daily intake of carbohydrates is only one part of the efficacy of a diet.

Will this diet cause gallstones?

Gallstones are common in obese people, and if you are very overweight, a high-fat diet might cause you to become symptomatic. But this diet should not cause gallstone formation.

Will low-carbohydrate dieting give me kidney disease?

No. There are no studies showing that a low-carbohydrate diet can actually cause kidney damage to healthy kidneys. If you already have kidney disease, you should talk to your doctor about how much protein you should eat each day regardless of what diet you follow.

Can the high oxalate levels found in some vegetables be harmful?

Some green vegetables, legumes, fruits, nuts, grains, chocolate, teas (including herbal teas), and spices are high in oxalic acid (oxalates).

Meats, fats, and dairy foods, on the other hand, have almost no oxalates.

If you are prone to getting oxalate kidney stones, you may be told to avoid high-oxalate foods. A nutritionist can give you a complete list of foods to avoid. These foods include berries, figs, kiwis, citrus peels, whole-wheat bread, wheat germ, high-bran cereals, wheat bran, oatmeal, tofu, beans, nuts, greens, celery, eggplant, leeks, broccoli, cauliflower, parsley, yellow squash, carrots, green beans, green peppers, tomatoes, yams, and chocolate.

Almost any balanced diet will include some of these nutritious foods, most of which would be recommended on the "eat more fruits and vegetables and less fat" diet that is currently popular with nutritionists. The meats and dairy products they recommend avoiding, on the other hand, are low in oxalates.

So what's the bottom line? Is this diet safe?
We think so. Ask any physician if it is safer to be thinner eating a low-carbohydrate diet or obese on a high-carbohydrate diet.

Exercise

Do I have to exercise?
Not until you can. Consult your physician.

Farmers' Markets

Where can I find a good farmers' market?
Look on the Web site of the municipality in which you live. Call the local chamber of commerce. In rural areas, agricultural groups usually publish lists of local farmers' markets as well as local farmers who have farm stands or pick-your-own businesses. If there's an extension service in your town, they should have lists of farmers' markets. Or ask your friends and coworkers.

Fiber

What is fiber?
Fiber is the indigestible carbohydrates of plants. Rich sources include nuts, vegetables, psyllium, brans, and flaxseeds.

Fruit

I love fruit, but I'm only allowed to eat a half cup of fruit a day. Any suggestions?

Yes. You can have only one serving of fruit a day, but you don't need to eat the whole serving at once. This is especially important if you have diabetes and find that, for example, a whole slice of melon makes your blood glucose levels go too high but you hate to give up melons.

Just measure out the whole fruit serving and eat a little bit of it with each meal. Yogurt is a great way to "stretch" the taste of fruit. A few berries stirred into yogurt make the whole yogurt serving taste like fruit with very few berries.

Growing Children

Is this diet okay for my growing children and teenagers?

In general, yes. There are no caloric restrictions so they should eat the amounts of good foods they require. It's healthy in that the basics of nutritional needs are ensured every day. The diet exposes them to a variety of foods (especially vegetables) and steers them away from high-saturated-fat and sugar- and starch-dense foods, which is good.

Headaches

Why do I get headaches?

Headaches are normal in the first two to three days as your body adjusts to the diet. After that it is usually a sign of dehydration. Drink more fluids.

Heavy Exercise

I run twenty miles a day. Does this affect how many carbs I can eat?

Seems like everyone exaggerates their exercise, doesn't it? If you do in fact exercise excessively—preparing for a marathon or similar event—you'll need to consult references for the type of nutrition that is needed. Caloric needs are high, and you should not follow any type of weight-reduction program simultaneously, as it may affect your muscle mass.

If you are a moderate exerciser—say, tennis once or twice week and daily walking, there should be no need to change the recommendations.

My son is on the football team. Does he need more carbs or just more food?

Your son should work with his coach or the team's trainer to determine his nutritional needs during the football season. An aggressive football training schedule combined with adolescent growth is beyond the scope of this book.

How Long?

How long must I stay on the Four Corners Diet?

As long as it takes. Never go back to what you are doing now. That's what got you into trouble. You should probably eat this way for the rest of your life. Don't think of it as a diet, though. Think of it as a healthy approach to eating.

Hunger

Will I be hungry?

Probably not. This diet produces natural hunger suppressants. Never go hungry. Eat low-carb snacks to tide you over.

Ketones

Is ketosis dangerous?

Ketosis is not necessarily dangerous. It is one measurement to show that your body is burning fat. You may lose weight (fat) without showing ketones in your urine, so we do not see any benefit to monitoring your urine with ketone test strips. Ketones in the urine is not your objective; weight loss is.

Is ketosis the same as ketoacidosis?

No. Ketoacidosis is a dangerous condition associated with type 1 diabetes.

Organic and Genetically Engineered Foods

Does it matter if I buy organic foods or not?

This is a controversial point. Even the definition of "organic" according to the U.S. Department of Agriculture seems to be changing. In general, try to buy fresh food from local producers, wash everything, peel what you can, and watch for more information on food standards as they develop.

How about genetically engineered foods?

This, too, is controversial. In Europe, they're not allowed. In the United States, they are. You may not even know if a food has been altered or not since the producer is not required to disclose.

Psyllium

What is psyllium?

It is the husk of a grass seed. Buy sugar-free flavored or plain Metamucil. Even better, buy the pure psyllium powders that have no maltodextrin as bulking agents. You can find pure psyllium at the drugstore or in health food stores.

Use it in wheat-bran pancakes and meatballs, or drink it in club soda. Guar gum or xanthan gum can also be used.

Recipes

Where can I find good recipes?

We've included enough recipes in this book to get you started. For more, look on the Internet and in bookstores for low-carbohydrate cookbooks. There are now a lot of such cookbooks, ranging from gourmet low-carb cooking to everyday low-carb cooking.

Just make sure the recipes don't exceed the limits of this diet: 15 grams of net carbohydrate per meal and 50 grams per day. Some low-carb recipes are low in carbohydrate compared with the average American diet but have too many carbohydrates for this way of eating.

Also, make sure the recipes in these cookbooks aren't too high in saturated fat.

Seek out others who are following this diet and exchange recipes with them, if possible.

Snacks

Are snacks allowed?

Yes, so long as they are low-carbohydrate snacks like chicken wings, jerky, cheese, macadamia nuts, low-carb veggies with dips, pork rinds, and hard-boiled eggs.

Soy

Are soy products good for this diet?

Yes, *but*—read every label very closely. Soy milk can contain 8 grams or 28 grams of carbohydrate per 8 ounces. Both are labeled as "soy milk." Read every label before deciding. There are now artificially sweetened and calcium-fortified soy milks on the marked (for example, Soy Slender).

Supplements

Should I take any supplements on this diet?

Postmenopausal women and vegans should take 500 milligrams to 1 gram of supplemental calcium daily. All adults are currently advised to take a daily general multivitamin and mineral supplement, regardless of their diet.

Triglycerides

Will all that fat increase my blood triglycerides?

No. Most high blood triglycerides are caused by carbohydrate inges-tion. Almost all people will lower their serum triglyceride levels when following the Four Corners Diet.

Vegetable Servings

You said one serving of a vegetable is a cup raw or a half cup cooked. For fresh broccoli, it's the same cooked or raw. How much should I eat?

It's hard when foods don't do what they're supposed to do, isn't it? Broccoli, cauliflower, and Brussels sprouts just won't allow themselves to be measured in a measuring cup. Fortunately, they're all so low in carbohydrates that eating according to the "raw" recommendations isn't a problem.

Vegetarianism

Can I be vegetarian?

Yes, you can. The Recipe section contains a number of vegetarian recipes.

Texturized soy protein can be substituted for meat in other recipes. If you are vegan, you can create yogurt from soy milk and use soy sub-stitutions for cheese.

Water

How much water should I drink?

We recommend six to eight glasses of water or other fluids a day. You can include small amounts of coffee (one or two cups a day) as part of your fluid, but if you drink more than that, it acts as a diuretic (makes you lose more fluid than you take in), so you'll have to drink extra water to compensate.

Weight Loss

How fast will I lose weight?

This varies for each individual and also depends on how strict you are at cutting carbohydrates. It may vary from one to three pounds per week after the initial rapid weight loss until you reach your target weight.

FIFTEEN

Shopping

THE TWO MOST difficult things at the beginning of the transition to eating on the Four Corners Diet are changing your mind-set and retooling your pantry. No doubt your household is filled with foods that are low-fat or fat-free. Ours certainly were.

When you stop to read the labels, it will become painfully obvious that many of the things in your kitchen cabinets and pantry are incompatible with life on your new diet. So let's start by looking at labels, and then we can clean your cupboards out.

■

THE NUTRITION FACTS LABEL

ON THE BACKS of every manufactured food sold will be a nutrition facts label (see Figure 15.1 on next page). This label starts by giving the serving size. For example, a "serving" may be defined as "7 crackers" or "1 ounce" or "2 slices." The "servings per container" will then be given. This is followed by "calories" and "calories from fat," which on this diet you can finally ignore. Next will be a table showing the "amount per serving" of total fat (subcategories of saturated fat and sometimes monounsaturated and polyunsaturated fats are given; in 2006 labels will be required to indicate the amount of trans fat), cholesterol, sodium, total carbohydrate (and the subcategories fiber and sugars), and protein.

TABLE 15.1
Sample Nutrition Facts Label
❖

Nutrition Facts
Serving Size 3 pieces (15g)
Servings Per Container 15

Amount Per Serving

Calories 60	Calories from Fat 25

	% Daily Value*
Total Fat 3g	5%
Saturated Fat 0.5g	3%
Polyunsaturated Fat 0.5g	
Monounsaturated Fat 1.0g	
Cholesterol 0mg	0%
Sodium 110mg	5%
Total Carbohydrate 9g	3%
Dietary Fiber 1g	4%
Sugars 0.5g	
Protein 2g	

Vitamin A 0%	•	Vitamin C 0%
Calcium 0%	•	Iron 4%

* Percent Daily Values are based on a 2,000 calorie diet. Your daily values may be higher or lower depending on your calorie needs:

	Calories:	2,000	2,500
Total Fat	Less than	65g	60g
Sat. Fat	Less than	20g	25g
Cholesterol	Less than	300mg	300mg
Sodium	Less than	2,400mg	2,400mg
Total Carbohydrate		300g	375g
Dietary Fiber		25g	30g

INGREDIENTS: UNBLEACHED ENRICHED WHEAT FLOUR [FLOUR, MALTED BARLEY, NIACIN, REDUCED IRON, THIAMIN, MONONITRATE (VITAMIN B1), RIBOFLAVIN (VITAMIN B2), FOLIC ACID], PARTIALLY HYDROGENATED SOYBEAN OIL, OAT FIBER, DEXTROSE, SALT, YEAST.

Let's look a little closer at the total carbohydrate and its subcategories. This is the part of the label that is absolutely critical to read first. It will immediately tell you if you can even consider this food or not.

As you well know by now, you are limited to a total daily *net* carbohydrate intake of 50 grams, with only 12 to 15 grams of *net* carbohydrate at any one meal. And *everything* that might enter your mouth must be looked at for its carbohydrate content, whether it's solid or liquid, whether it's the meal or the dessert, whether it's the main course or a condiment, whether it's eaten standing up or sitting down. You get the picture.

Total carbohydrates per serving gives you the total grams of sugars, starches, and fiber in that particular serving size of that particular food. In Figure 15.1 this would be 9 grams. However, in the subdivisions below the total, often only the fiber and sugar content are shown, and not the starch. The product shown in Figure 15.1 has 1 gram of fiber and a half a gram of sugar. If these two are added together (1.5 grams) and then subtracted from the total, the remainder (7.5 grams) will be starches.

Now we told you earlier that fiber is "free." You don't have to count fiber in your total carbohydrate count. So, *subtract the grams of fiber from the total carbohydrate* shown in order to get the *net* carbohydrates, which is the number we are interested in (see page 15 to review).

Net carbohydrates are the starches and sugars in that serving size of the food in question. The product shown in Figure 15.1 has 8 grams of net carbs per 3 pieces (15 grams). The net carbohydrate is the amount that you are concerned with, the amount that must be counted into your carbohydrate allowance for that meal.

Now you can decide if it's possible for you to eat that food or to use that product in your food preparation. How many grams are left? Are you willing to use your carbohydrate allowance for that meal on that food? Or, when all the math is done, is the result so high that you just can't eat any? You may be surprised to find that a lot of the processed foods in your old pantry meet that "just can't eat any" category.

Take a minute now and look at some of the food products in your pantry. Cereals made from milled flours often have carbohydrate counts that exceed the limit, so these will probably be out. But if you have a cereal with a very high fiber level, it may be okay. Do the math to find out. Cookie carbohydrate counts are obviously in excess. Check out the package labels for rice and couscous. The answer is the same: too high. Pretzels, rice cakes, snack crackers, potato chips and sticks, and low-fat snacks? Again, too many net carbs. Time to clean house. Don't feel bad. These things were driving your weight gain. They *need* to go. If you feel bad about throwing away unopened high-carb foods, give them to a neighbor or donate them to a food bank.

So, processed foods will have to be carefully scrutinized before you buy anything. What's left to eat? Natural foods will have a better chance of working. Let's take another look at Table 4.2 to get a feel for the net carbohydrate count of many unprocessed foods. Which foods look like good choices, and which do not?

One caveat: in this table, and in any other carbohydrate counters that you may consult, be sure to pay attention to the serving size. In some cases, the serving size may represent more or less than what you would usually eat. For example, in Table 4.2 the serving size for heavy cream is 1 cup, which has 6.7 grams of carbs. Most people would never eat a cup of heavy cream at one sitting. Hence you must multiply or divide accordingly to adjust for what size you would *actually* eat. In this case, the amount of heavy cream you'd put in your coffee or whip to put on gelatin dessert would have less than 1 gram of carbs.

In Table 4.2 we selected many foods that are low in net carbohydrates, even with very generous serving sizes. This list is a good place to start to pick out foods for your shopping list. You'll notice that potatoes, sweet potatoes, rice, pasta, peas, corn, pretzels, bagels, and bread are *not* listed. Let's try to find substitutes for these foods from the approved foods (see also Chapter 7).

SHOPPING DAY

CAREFUL SHOPPING IS important. If you have your supplies on hand, you will be less tempted to break the diet.

Start out with a shopping list. The following food lists are a good place to start; later you can modify and expand according to your tastes. The Four Corners Diet will not feel like previous diets. You will notice that the foods you will be eating are not "hardships." They are really good foods that you may have been avoiding. Let's take a look.

Condiments

Mustard, horseradish, real mayonnaise, soy sauce, iodized salt, pepper, a variety of cooking spices, spray and liquid canola oil, olive oil, salsa without sugar, guacamole, sugar-free no-calorie gelatin, sugar-free (diabetic) syrups.

Vegetables

Mixed greens, lettuce, radishes, onions, celery, cucumbers, collards, okra, green beans, wax beans, spinach, zucchini, spaghetti squash, summer squash, acorn squash, cauliflower, broccoli, Brussels sprouts, mushrooms, mixed Chinese vegetables.

You can buy these fresh or frozen or canned—provided there are no added sugars. Buy plenty of variety and amount, because you are expected to have five servings of vegetables a day. A serving size is roughly 1 cup of the raw vegetable or ½ cup cooked.

Meats and Fish

Fresh, unbreaded, lean poultry, beef, veal, pork. Fresh fish and shellfish. Canned tuna, salmon, and sardines in oil or water. Low-saturated-fat sausages and prepared luncheon meats. Remember to check that there are no added fillers in the sausages or meats. If you're vegetarian, check out soy and veggie burgers.

Fruits

Buy a *very* limited amount of fresh, unsweetened berries, kiwis, rhubarb, or melons or low-sugar tart apples or pears. Avoid frozen berries unless you are sure there is no sugar or syrup added. Remember your serving size is only ½ cup of *one* of these per day. Don't overbuy.

Dairy/Eggs/Cheese

Cultured, fermented milk products should be first on your list because we encourage 8 ounces of kefir, buttermilk, or yogurt daily.

Cheese blocks or cubes, string cheese, ricotta cheese, cream cheese, eggs, and heavy cream. If you read labels closely, you may be able to find artificially sweetened yogurt without fruit that will be okay.

THE TWO FACES OF FISH

Most fish are healthy foods, because they contain a lot of the beneficial omega-3 fatty acids. You may have heard that you should focus especially on the fatty cold-water fish such as salmon and mackerel.

Today, however, with the increasing pollution in the world, fatty fish also accumulate harmful toxins, including mercury and PCBs. In addition, some of the farmed fish such as salmon are fed commercial grains and artificial dyes and may have different nutritional profiles than wild fish.

Toxins accumulate in fatty tissues and tend to stay there for the lifetime of the animal. If another animal eats it, the toxins get absorbed by the eater. The larger the fish, the higher on the food chain and the greater the possibility of accumulating toxins. Hence the big fish like tuna, swordfish, and salmon are the most likely to be contaminated (and polar bears are said to be one of the most contaminated organisms on earth).

Wild fish tend to be healthier than farmed, but if everyone ate only wild fish, the world's fish stocks would become depleted even more rapidly than they are already.

So what should you do? Are fish healthy or are fish harmful? The answer is both.

One solution is to eat a variety of fish, so if any variety has accumulated a particular toxin, you won't get too much of that. Another is to focus on the smaller fish like sardines, which are closer to the bottom of the food chain. Don't go overboard with the large fatty fish. And when you do eat fish, make sure it's the best quality you can afford.

Cereal/Crackers

Look very closely and don't get tricked by the labels. You *can* find extremely high-fiber bran cereal and high-fiber, low-net-carbohydrate crispbread. Low-carb breads and tortillas are now available at some health food stores and more are appearing in regular grocery stores every day.

Buy wheat or rice bran and flaxseed. You may have to look especially hard at first to find these, but it will be worth your effort for cooking your own pancakes and waffles and cereals.

Nuts and Seeds

Pecans, almonds, macadamias, hazelnuts, walnuts, peanuts, and edible seeds such as pumpkin seeds and sunflower seed kernels. Find the ones you like and buy them in bulk by the pound at wholesale stores for the freshest product and best prices. Avoid chestnuts and cashews, which contain more carbs. Brazil nuts and pistachios are fine as part of a mixed nuts assortment, but it's best not to eat them alone. Brazil nuts contain more saturated fats than other nuts, and pistachios contain more carbohydrates.

Drinks

Kefir, diet soda, diet powdered drinks, tea, coffee, light beer or dry wine, diet-only mixers, kefir or yogurt shakes, and smoothies.

What about those packaged foods that we've all become so dependent upon for convenience? Well, sadly, many of those foods are excessively high in carbohydrate counts. When we need convenience, we have to start thinking differently. For example, think "rotisserie chicken and salad" instead of "frozen pizza." Both are available at most larger grocery stores. You just have to look at the deli sections now instead of the frozen-food sections. Snacks become nuts and cheese instead of pretzels and rice cakes. No cookies or candy; instead buy sugar-free, flavored gelatin for use alone or with sugar-free whipped topping. No breakfast tarts or premade waffles. Instead, substitute high-fiber crispbread with cream cheese and wheat-bran waffles that you can make in advance and freeze, then pop in the toaster or microwave.

It may seem hard at first, but that is part of the education and retooling process. You have to make new, healthy eating habits replace the old habits that gave rise to an unhealthy (and overweight) lifestyle. Once you have the proper ingredients and assortment of the right foods in the house, it's a lot easier.

SIXTEEN

Menu Suggestions

I N PREVIOUS CHAPTERS we supplied you with seven days of menus to get you started. The Recipe section provides many delicious recipes that work for the Four Corners Diet.

But the most difficult part of any new diet is menu planning, and you may still want a little help in that area, so we have provided here a few more suggestions for healthy meals.

Remember, menu planning is the key to success. You need to organize your shopping and menu planning so you will have the proper ingredients on hand to prepare enjoyable food that will help you stick with this way of eating.

You don't want to fall into old habits when you get to the store. So sit down and plan what you will eat for the next week. Then make sure you have all the necessary ingredients available.

Rediscover some great kitchen cooking aids: the slow cooker, the pressure cooker, and the electric skillet. Undoubtedly you have them hidden somewhere in the pantry. These can be lifesavers for the hectic household and will help you avoid convenience foods.

Here are a few inexpensive kitchen gadgets that will make your life much easier:

- ❖ A waffle iron
- ❖ A yogurt incubator
- ❖ A good blender with a heavy-duty motor. Making smoothies and cheesecakes and pumpkin pies is easy when your blender can handle the task.
- ❖ A pressure cooker
- ❖ A slow cooker
- ❖ An electric skillet
- ❖ An ice cream maker (yes, it's allowed if you make it with real cream or if you make your own frozen yogurt)

And here are a few menu ideas to get you started:

FOR THE SLOW COOKER

- ❖ Start a pot roast with leeks, carrots, and celery in the morning and come home to a house filled with savory fragrances. Use a gravy enhancer, concentrated beef seasoning, and your favorite spices. Remember, in a slow cooker, keep liquids to a minimum.
- ❖ Start chili with 2 pounds of prebrowned ground beef, chopped onions, celery, and green pepper, 1 can of crushed tomatoes, and chili seasonings to taste. Let it cook all day in the slow cooker and dress it up with shredded cheese, sour cream, and guacamole when you serve it.
- ❖ Put lean Italian sausages in the slow cooker. Cover with a few tablespoons of low-carb seasoned tomato sauce or crushed tomatoes. Top with sliced onions and green pepper. Cook on "low" all day. Serve with spaghetti squash. Top with shredded mozzarella.
- ❖ Make a sausage stew as above, but cut up the Italian sausages into quarters and add loads of mushrooms, celery, onions, and zucchini slices in with the sausage and tomato sauce. Serve with Parmesan sprinkled over the stew.

FOR THE ELECTRIC SKILLET
(THINK MORE ONE-DISH MEALS)

❖ Pull out some boneless chicken breasts and sauté in olive oil with garlic. Add sliced eggplant, zucchini, onions, green peppers, and more olive oil, and cook until done. Add salt and pepper and enjoy a skillet dinner in minutes.

❖ Sauté beef fillets in oil. Cover and cook through to desired doneness. Remove from the skillet to a plate. Now add more oil and sauté sliced onions, green peppers, and mushrooms. Put these on your beef. Steam assorted vegetables, and dinner is served.

FOR THE PRESSURE COOKER

❖ Try Dr. Goldberg's favorite chicken soup recipe in the pressure cooker and create a classic dish in a fraction of the time.

❖ Make a stew in minutes.

❖ Buy the cheapest cuts of meat and make them taste like expensive cuts.

❖ Prepare a vegetable mushroom soup. Add cream just before serving.

BREAKFASTS

BREAKFASTS CAN BE varied. All breakfasts can be served with coffee or tea. Try the following:

❖ Two large eggs in butter/olive oil mixture with 1 ounce of Swiss cheese; 1 cup of plain kefir, plain or artificially sweetened to taste

❖ Wheat-bran waffles topped with strawberries; with lean sausage

❖ Ricotta cheese pancakes

❖ Yogurt, artificially sweetened and mixed with chopped pecans and cinnamon

Menu Suggestions

- Bacon and eggs along with high-fiber crispbread and peanut butter
- Smoked fish, cheese slices, high-fiber crispbread, and yogurt
- Fried steak and onions and high-fiber crispbread
- High-fiber crispbreads with peanut butter or cream cheese, lox, tomato, capers, and onions
- Chopped tomatoes, chopped cucumbers, and sprouts dressed with olive oil and tuna or smoked fish
- String cheese, mixed nuts, and coffee in a cup to go when you're on the run to the train
- Easy "eggs Benedict": poach an egg and serve on a slice of ham with lemon and olive oil
- Breakfast parfait with layers of plain yogurt, mixed fresh berries, high-fiber bran cereal

LUNCHES

- Tuna salad made with real mayonnaise and pickle relish and hard-boiled eggs (use 1 6-ounce can of tuna per person); tossed salad with olive oil vinaigrette
- One can of sardines packed in olive oil mashed with a hard-boiled egg; cucumber slices; 1 ounce of macadamia or other nuts-and-seeds mixture
- Deviled eggs, cheddar cheese, and cucumber slices
- Grilled chicken breast; multi-vegetable tossed salad with olive oil vinaigrette
- Double cheeseburger (no bun); tossed salad with olive oil vinaigrette
- Half a cold roast chicken; broccoli salad with onions and cheese
- Egg salad; tossed salad with olive oil vinaigrette
- Grilled or pan-fried or baked fish; steamed assorted vegetables
- Reheated leftovers from last night's dinner
- Two Polish or Italian sausages; sauerkraut; tossed salad
- Crustless quiche, tossed salad with oil and vinegar; steamed vegetables
- Hearty vegetable beef soup and tossed salad

■

DINNER

- ❖ Vegetable consommé; roast chicken with mashed cauliflower; tossed salad with olive oil vinaigrette; small slice of artificially sweetened pumpkin pie made with a nut crust and served with whipped cream
- ❖ Large steak, trimmed lean; fried onions; stir-fried zucchini; tossed salad with olive oil vinaigrette; ½ cup strawberries and cream
- ❖ Eggplant Parmesan ("bread" the eggplant with wheat bran and proceed with usual recipe); tossed salad with olive oil vinaigrette; blueberry and yogurt smoothie
- ❖ Pork roast; acorn squash with butter and garlic; collard greens or creamed spinach; melon
- ❖ Vegetable soufflé; tossed salad with olive oil vinaigrette; sugar-free flavored gelatin and whipped cream
- ❖ All-meat (check to make sure they don't contain carbohydrate fillers) hot dogs or bratwurst; sauerkraut; dill pickles; tossed salad with olive oil vinaigrette
- ❖ Chicken and vegetable stir-fry on a bed of "riced" cauliflower; sugar-free cheesecake
- ❖ Meatballs and tomato sauce with spaghetti squash; tossed salad with olive oil vinaigrette; flavored coffee and real cream
- ❖ Deli meats and chopped liver; homemade coleslaw and pickles; crispbread and crispy lettuce leaves to wrap meat
- ❖ Pot roast with leeks, carrots, celery; mashed cauliflower; salad
- ❖ Grilled or baked fish; steamed broccoli and cauliflower; sautéed mushrooms
- ❖ Roast turkey; grated zucchini and sausage stuffing; steamed vegetables; salad; rhubarb crisp (topping made with ground nuts and bran) served with whipped cream
- ❖ Shish kabob with shrimp, scallops, chicken, and vegetables; tossed salad with olive oil vinaigrette; root beer float made with cream and diet root beer
- ❖ Grilled burgers, ribs, steaks, just about anything made on the grill provided you make your own barbecue sauce that is sweetened artificially. Try grilled vegetables seasoned with sugar-free Italian dressing

Menu Suggestions

❖ Upside-down pizza. Coat a glass ovenproof dish with canola or olive oil. Build an upside-down pizza as follows. *Bottom layer:* sliced Italian sausage or pepperoni. *Next layer:* sliced mushrooms, chopped spinach, sliced onions, peppers, and other toppings. *Next layer:* sprinkle of oregano, crushed garlic, and crushed red peppers to taste. Finally, top with a generous layer of mozzarella or mixed, shredded pizza cheeses. Bake at 400°F until the top melts and browns. Serve straight from the dish.

■

SNACKS

❖ Nuts and seeds
❖ Kefir and yogurt smoothies
❖ Chicken legs or wings roasted and dipped into a variety of no- or low-carbohydrate condiments
❖ No-bake artificially sweetened cheesecakes, sugar-free pumpkin pie, strawberries, floats made from heavy cream, and diet pop
❖ Hard salami slices and deli meats (look for lean varieties and use in moderation), cheese of all types, pork rinds
❖ Hard-boiled and deviled eggs
❖ Fresh vegetables dipped in guacamole or salsa
❖ High-fiber crispbread with peanut butter or cream cheese or sour cream "chip" dips
❖ Flavored coffees and cream
❖ Peanut butter spread on garden vegetables, for example, crispy fresh green peppers

■

DESSERTS

❖ Artificially sweetened, flavored yogurts
❖ Homemade frozen yogurt
❖ Flavored diet soda with 1 to 2 ounces of heavy cream, or flavored coffees with a dollop of whipped cream
❖ Assortment of cheeses and nuts

❖ Sugar-free flavored gelatin with berries

❖ High-fiber crispbread and flavored cream cheese

❖ Artificially sweetened chopped rhubarb with a crisp crust of crushed nuts, bran, artificial brown sugar, and butter "crisped" in the oven

❖ Dessert soufflé with granulated sugar substitute when you're feeling energetic and enthusiastic about cooking

❖ A package of instant, sugar-free pudding mixed with kefir instead of milk when you're feeling too pooped to cook

By now, you probably have a good idea of how to create menus. You eat good food and make choices from the many low-carbohydrate items that you are now getting accustomed to thinking about. Stretch your memory and try to think of home cooking from your childhood. Many of those foods—for example, hearty homemade soups and stews (just minus the potatoes and dumplings)—are fine for this diet.

In the summer, grill meats and fish on the backyard grill. Keep coleslaw or broccoli slaw in the refrigerator for side dishes. Slice vegetables and marinade in seasoned oil and vinegar or lemon, and then throw these on the grill, too. Dress chopped onions, green peppers, and tomatoes with oil and vinegar, salt, and pepper, and keep in a covered container in the refrigerator for a healthy side salad. Be creative with vegetables. Construct a bacon, lettuce, and tomato salad.

In cold weather, use your slow cooker and make pot roast, chilis, and stews. In general, you should avoid beans and lentils. But for a special treat, you can make a low-bean chili. Use only one can of kidney beans to a full pot of chili so that the carbohydrate count will be low per serving size. Even better: use black soybeans. They have a lower carb count, and you probably won't notice the difference. Add celery for more texture and fiber. Top with chopped onions, green pepper, shredded cheese, and guacamole. Put a small pot roast or boneless pork roast in a slow cooker, cover with salsa, and cook on "low" all day. When you get home, shred the meat and turn it into a taco salad by putting the meat on a bed of lettuce and topping it with sour cream, guacamole, cheese, and salsa.

Can you have a turkey dinner? Of course. Be sure to trim that roasted turkey with mashed cauliflower, asparagus and cheese sauce, mixed green salad, and baked acorn squash. You can make a good cranberry sauce by adding chopped fresh cranberries and walnuts to sugar-free orange gelatin. Missing anything? Make a sugar-free pumpkin pie with whipped cream.

Can you make a breakfast on the run? Of course. Pack up nuts and string cheese to eat on the train. Or maybe crispbread and peanut butter. Try a kefir shake.

Note that because of the increasing popularity of low-carbohydrate diets, increasing numbers of low-carb meal-replacement foods such as bars and shakes are now available. Buyer beware. Many of these products have little nutritional value, and some contain harmful trans fats and hidden carbs. They may come in handy in an emergency, when there's nothing else to eat. But don't be tempted to make them part of your regular routine when you're in a hurry. Remember, there are four corners to this diet. Real, whole foods are what you want, not candy bars.

Now review the list of menu suggestions. There are a lot of choices. Menu planning should be getting easier. The Recipe section will get you started, but remember, you can adapt many of your favorite recipes, too.

Once you break out of your old eating patterns and switch to really good, healthy foods, you'll be glad you decided to embark on the Four Corners way of eating.

▶ IF YOU HAVE DIABETES

STEWS AND SLOW-COOKER recipes are great time-savers, especially when you work all day and come home exhausted. However, you should be aware that long cooking tends to break down the fiber in vegetables and may increase their glycemic index values.

So when you try a recipe that includes a lot of vegetables, make sure to use your meter to test after you eat that meal so you'll know if it's okay for you. If not, you may want to reduce the content of some of the higher-carb vegetables such as carrots, leeks, onions, and tomatoes.

Your meter puts you in charge. Use it.

SEVENTEEN

Recipes

EATING THE FOUR CORNERS way doesn't have to be a dull regimen of meat and salad. Once you learn how to use vegetables, high-fiber brans and breads, and yogurt and kefir in place of the processed grains, breads, oversweet fruit juices, and milk that you've used in the past, a whole new world of delicious recipes and new tastes will open up to you.

Following is a selection of recipes to get you started. We've used these recipes in our homes, and we find them practical as well as healthy. Most of them use ordinary ingredients and won't require you to scour your city for unusual vegetables or spices. Most can be prepared in a reasonable amount of time, an important aspect for the home cook in today's busy world.

We hope you will go beyond these recipes and create wonderful-tasting Four Corners dishes of your own, based on your own ethnic heritage and family recipes, adapting them to be low in carbohydrates and high in fiber, monounsaturated fat, probiotics, and pharmafoods.

Think about food values. Plan to add fresh vegetables to all your meal planning. Think about fiber, and look for ways to add wheat or rice bran or psyllium husks. Think about crushed nuts or high-fiber crispbread as substitutes for graham cracker crusts.

Many of your favorite recipes can be made low carbohydrate by substituting no-calorie sweeteners for sugar, and cream or kefir for milk. Use wheat or rice bran, soy flour, and soy powder in place of milled white or wheat flour.

For instance, you can use the famous canned pumpkin pie recipe by substituting granulated sugar substitute for sugar, and cream or kefir for condensed milk. A ground-nut crust can be made instead of the conventional pie crust. In fact, many find the nut crusts to be superior to the traditional graham cracker crusts for pies.

How about other fillings? You could fill that crust with your favorite quiche recipe. It fits perfectly into the Four Corners way of eating. Quiche can also be made entirely crustless. Soufflés also fit well into the Four Corners Diet.

Your favorite cheesecake recipe is likewise adaptable to such substitutions. Except for the sugar, everything else in a cheesecake recipe is legal if you use a nut crust in place of graham crackers. Just take your favorite recipe, substitute a granulated no-calorie sugar substitute, and bake as usual.

Many cookbooks can help you. For instance, vegetable and egg cookbooks offer a variety of selections. Make sugar substitutions with no-calorie sweeteners when appropriate. There is even a brown sugar substitute.

Most meat, fish, and egg recipes can be made low carbohydrate with little trouble. Look in French-style cookbooks for sauces and foods that are usually low carbohydrate.

The recipes provided here include the net carbohydrate and the percentage of monounsaturated fat for each ingredient as well as for the recipe as a whole (more deetailed nutritional analyses are provided in Appendix II, pages 216–231). With experience you should be able to calculate net carbs and estimate the amount of monounstaturated fat in your own recipes.

Don't panic. Many of your favorite recipes can be used without any changes, especially soups, stews, and casseroles with cheeses and eggs. Watch out for corn, peas, beans, and potatoes in these recipes and either eliminate them or substitute an approved vegetable.

Very soon you will be eating to live, not living to eat. And you won't miss the tasteless high-starch foods you had been eating.

Get involved with the diet. Read as much as you can. Try recipes. Make the commitment. For those who have Internet capabilities, do a search on low-carbohydrate dieting. Just don't go overboard with the saturated fat that is found in some of the recipes on these sites. Join newsgroups. Make friends with others who are your kindred spirits in this endeavor.

Most of all, good luck with your diet. Others have done it. You can do it, too.

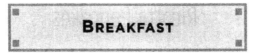

BREAKFAST

Baked French Toast with Apples

YIELD IS 6 SERVINGS, SERVING SIZE IS 1 SERVING

INGREDIENT	CARBS, GRAMS	FIBER, GRAMS	NET CARBS	% MONO
6 slices low-carb high-fiber bread*	24.0	6.0	18.0	*
2 Granny Smith apples	38.0	4.8	33.2	–
6 eggs	3.6	0.0	3.6	38
½ cup half-and-half (or milk)	7.8	0.0	7.8	29
6 packets sugar substitute (not aspartame)	5.4	0.0	5.4	–
1 teaspoon cinnamon	1.8	1.2	0.6	–
RECIPE TOTAL	80.6	12.0	68.6	*
SERVING TOTAL (rounded)	13	2	11	*

* There are many different low-carb breads on the market, and they differ in their carb content. This analysis used the Food for Life brand. This product, with 4 grams of fat per slice, does not list the amount of monounsaturated fat. The label says there are zero grams of saturated fat.

1. Spray-oil a 13- x 9-inch baking pan. Place bread slices on the bottom to form a layer.
2. Peel and slice apples thinly and layer slices on top of bread. Whisk together eggs and remaining ingredients. Pour over the bread and apples. Cover pan with cling wrap and refrigerate overnight.
3. Next morning, bake at 350°F for 50–60 minutes until puffed and browned.
4. Cut into serving portions and serve with sugar-free syrup or cooked berries, sweetened with sugar substitute as desired.

▶ Makes 6 to 8 servings
▶ Excellent breakfast or brunch dish
▶ Serve with lean bacon or sausage on the side for a substantive meal.
▶ See page 216 for more detailed nutrient contents per serving.

Ricotta Pancakes

YIELD IS 6 SERVINGS, SERVING SIZE IS 1 PANCAKE

INGREDIENT	CARBS, GRAMS	FIBER, GRAMS	NET CARBS	% MONO
8 ounces ricotta cheese	7.5	0.0	7.5	66
1 tablespoon olive oil	0.0	0.0	0.0	73
½ cup almond flour (ground almonds)	9.7	5.2	4.5	65
2 large eggs	2.4	0.0	2.4	38
1 packet sugar substitute (not aspartame)	0.9	0.0	0.9	—
1 teaspoon vanilla	0.5	0.0	0.5	—
Pinch of salt	0.0	0.0	0.0	—
3 tablespoons canola oil for frying	0.0	0.0	0.0	60
RECIPE TOTAL	21.0	5.2	15.8	51
SERVING TOTAL (rounded)	4	1	3	51

1. Mix all ingredients but canola oil until batter is smooth. Add canola oil to a crepe pan. Add heat to moderately hot. Add a few tablespoons of batter to pan. Swirl the pan to spread the batter.
2. Cook on the first side until bubbly and brown around the edges. Cook until firm. Then turn gently and fry until done.

▶ Makes 6 to 8 pancakes

▶ These are very thin pancakes, like crepes or blintzes

▶ If you can't find almond meal, you can substitute any other nut meal you can find, or you can grind your own from unsalted nuts.

▶ See page 216 for more detailed nutrient contents per serving.

Cheese Omelet

YIELD IS 1 SERVING, SERVING SIZE IS 1 SERVING

INGREDIENT	CARBS, GRAMS	FIBER, GRAMS	NET CARBS	% MONO
2 large eggs	1.2	0.0	1.2	38
2 tablespoons heavy cream	0.8	0.0	0.8	29
¼ teaspoon salt	0.0	0.0	0.0	—
¼ cup grated cheddar cheese (1 ounce)	0.4	0.0	0.4	29
1 tablespoon butter	0.0	0.0	0.0	29
1 tablespoon olive oil	0.0	0.0	0.0	73
RECIPE TOTAL	2.4	0.0	2.4	41
SERVING TOTAL (rounded)	2	0	2	41

1. Beat together the eggs, cream, and salt. Heat the pan and melt the butter. Add the oil. Lower the heat to medium and add the egg mixture.
2. Using a spatula, keep pushing the edge of the egg mixture toward the center of the pan, allowing the liquid center egg to flow back out. Work your way around the pan. When the omelet is almost cooked, sprinkle the cheese over half the pan.
3. Ease the omelet onto a plate. When it is halfway out of the pan, fold it over onto itself.

▶ Makes 1 omelet
▶ Variation: Use Swiss or other cheeses instead of cheddar.
▶ Variation: Use raw chopped vegetables, sautéed vegetables, or smoked salmon instead of cheese.
▶ A good omelet pan is essential for the best results. If you don't have one, you can use a regular frying pan, but the right tool for the job is a great help.
▶ See page 217 for more detailed nutrient contents per serving.

Fast Bran Cereal

YIELD IS 2 SERVINGS, SERVING SIZE IS 1 SERVING

INGREDIENT	CARBS, GRAMS	FIBER, GRAMS	NET CARBS	% MONO
¼ cup oat bran	15.6	3.6	12.0	35
¼ cup wheat bran	9.4	6.2	3.2	–
2 tablespoons flaxseed, freshly ground	8.2	6.7	1.5	20
1½ cups water	0.0	0.0	0.0	–
Pinch of salt (optional)	–	–	–	–
Sugar substitute to taste (not aspartame)	–	–	–	–
RECIPE TOTAL	33.2	16.5	16.7	22
SERVING TOTAL (rounded)	16	8	8	22

1. Mix all ingredients together in a microwave container. Microwave on high for 2½ minutes (cereal must heat to boiling). Let stand additional 1 minute.

▶ Makes 2 servings

▶ Variation: For even lower carb count, omit oat bran. For each serving, combine 2 tablespoons wheat bran and 2 tablespoons freshly ground flaxseed and ¼ to ⅔ cup boiling water and mix.

▶ Serve with walnuts and sunflower seeds.

▶ Top with cream or soy milk.

▶ Premix dry ingredients and store in baggies in the refrigerator for extra convenience in the morning.

▶ This is good with cinnamon, which is a pharmafood for people with diabetes.

▶ See page 217 for more detailed nutrient contents per serving.

Quick Bran Pancakes

YIELD IS 1 SERVING, SERVING SIZE IS 1 LARGE PANCAKE

INGREDIENT	CARBS, GRAMS	FIBER, GRAMS	NET CARBS	% MONO
2 eggs	1.2	0.0	1.2	38
4 tablespoons wheat bran	10.9	7.7	3.2	–
1 tablespoon psyllium seed husks	3.3	3.0	0.3	–
¼ teaspoon baking soda	0.0	0.0	0.0	–
1 tablespoon canola oil	0.0	0.0	0.0	60
1 packet sugar substitute (not aspartame)	0.9	0.0	0.9	–
RECIPE TOTAL	16.3	10.7	5.6	49
SERVING TOTAL (rounded)	16	11	6	49

1. Mix with a fork just before frying; otherwise, the psyllium will swell too much and make the pancake too gelatinous. Fry in oil and serve with sweetened kefir or yogurt.

▶ Makes 1 large or 2 small pancakes

▶ To make waffles, add the oil to the batter and cook in a waffle iron.

▶ Suggested flavorings for the kefir/yogurt: vanilla, maple, cinnamon, banana, or pureed berries. Use your imagination.

▶ Other topping suggestions: sour cream, 1 strawberry mashed in 2 tablespoons water and sweetened to taste.

▶ For a special treat add chopped pecans, walnuts, or almonds.

▶ You can use other brans if you're allergic to wheat. Rice bran has the fewest carbs of the brans available retail. You can also use different soluble fibers such as guar gum.

▶ Omit the baking powder if you're on a low-salt diet. The pancakes will still be delicious, although slightly less fluffy.

▶ For quick breakfasts, make a batch of pancakes and put the extras in the freezer. Then just defrost and eat.

▶ See page 217 for more detailed nutrient contents per serving.

Flax-Bran Pancakes

YIELD IS 1 SERVING, SERVING SIZE IS 1 LARGE PANCAKE

INGREDIENT	CARBS, GRAMS	FIBER, GRAMS	NET CARBS	%MONO
2 eggs	1.2	0.0	1.2	38
2 tablespoons wheat bran	5.5	3.8	1.7	–
4 tablespoons flaxseed, freshly ground	16.4	13.4	3.0	20
¼ teaspoon baking soda	0.0	0.0	0.0	–
1 packet sugar substitute (not aspartame)	0.9	0.0	0.9	–
12 blueberries	2.3	0.4	1.9	–
1 tablespoon canola oil	0.0	0.0	0.0	60
RECIPE TOTAL	26.3	17.6	8.7	38
SERVING TOTAL (rounded)	26	18	9	38

1. Mix with a fork just before frying; otherwise, the flax will swell too much and make it too gelatinous.
2. Fry in canola oil, turning pancake when you see air bubbles in the middle. Serve with sweetened kefir flavored with maple or vanilla (or other flavors) as a dipping sauce.

▶ **Makes 1 large or 2 small pancakes**
▶ **See page 217 for more detailed nutrient contents per serving.**

APPETIZERS AND SNACKS

Smoked Salmon Cheese Spread

YIELD IS 8 SERVINGS, SERVING SIZE IS 1 SERVING

INGREDIENT	CARBS, GRAMS	FIBER, GRAMS	NET CARBS	% MONO
1-pound can of salmon	0.0	0.0	0.0	35
1 pound cream cheese	12.1	0.0	12.1	28
¼ cup onions, chopped finely	3.5	0.7	2.8	–
1 teaspoon liquid smoke	–	–	–	–
Salt and pepper to taste	–	–	–	–
RECIPE TOTAL	15.5	0.7	14.8	29
SERVING TOTAL (rounded)	2	0	2	29

1. Blend salmon and cream cheese. Add onion and liquid smoke. Add salt and pepper to taste. Blend with large fork or spoon until smooth.
2. Serve with celery sticks, cucumber slices, other raw veggies, or high-fiber crispbreads.

▶ Makes 8 to 16 servings
▶ This is yummy for a party.
▶ Remember to add the carbs in the crispbreads if you eat them.
▶ See page 218 for more detailed nutrient contents per serving.

Blue Cheese Dip

YIELD IS 16 SERVINGS, SERVING SIZE IS 1 TABLESPOON

INGREDIENT	CARBS, GRAMS	FIBER, GRAMS	NET CARBS	% MONO
½ cup mayonnaise	2.4	0.0	2.4	27*
½ cup crumbled blue cheese	1.6	0.0	1.6	27
RECIPE TOTAL	4.0	0.0	4.0	27
SERVING TOTAL (rounded)	0	0	0	27

* Analysis is for standard commercial mayonnaise made with soybean oil, which is rich in polyunsaturates. To increase the percentage of monounsaturated fat, use homemade mayonnaise (72 percent mono fat) or commercial canola mayonnaise.

1. Mix cheese and mayonnaise together. Put into a bowl as a dip for mixed vegetables such as:

   Broccoli florets
   Cauliflower florets
   Cucumber slices
   Whole white mushrooms
   Celery sticks
   Zucchini and yellow squash slices

▶ **Makes 16 servings**
▶ **Variation: Use plain yogurt instead of mayonnaise.**
▶ **Easy party appetizer**
▶ **See page 218 for more detailed nutrient contents per serving.**

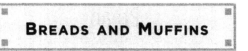

BREADS AND MUFFINS

Blueberry Muffins

YIELD IS 12 SERVINGS, SERVING SIZE IS 1 MUFFIN

INGREDIENT	CARBS, GRAMS	FIBER, GRAMS	NET CARBS	% MONO
5 large eggs	3.0	0.0	3.0	38
1 teaspoon baking powder	1.1	0.0	1.1	—
1 teaspoon vanilla extract	0.5	0.0	0.5	—
½ teaspoon lemon extract	—	—	—	—
1 cup sucralose (Splenda)	22.6	0.0	22.6	—
2 cups ground almonds (or any nut flour)	37.5	22.4	15.1	64
¾ cup canola oil	0.0	0.0	0.0	60
¼ teaspoon salt	0.0	0.0	0.0	—
½ cup blueberries	10.2	2.0	8.2	—
RECIPE TOTAL	74.9	24.4	50.5	59
SERVING TOTAL (rounded)	6	2	4	59

1. Preheat oven to 350°F.
2. Mix all ingredients except blueberries together with a large spoon until smooth.
3. Spoon into muffin paper baking cups in a muffin tin and add 4 or 5 blueberries to each muffin.
4. Bake for 30 minutes.

▶ Makes 12 muffins
▶ Variation: Pour batter into a 9-inch cake pan. After baking, allow to cool. Then slice in half and put strawberries and whipped cream between the layers. Serve as a birthday cake or just as a scrumptious dessert.
▶ See page 218 for more detailed nutrient contents per serving.

Bread

YIELD IS 6 SERVINGS, SERVING SIZE IS 1 SLICE

INGREDIENT	CARBS, GRAMS	FIBER, GRAMS	NET CARBS	% MONO
4 eggs	2.4	0.0	2.4	40
¼ cup club soda	0.0	0.0	0.0	–
¼ teaspoon salt	0.0	0.0	0.0	–
4 tablespoons mayonnaise	1.2	0.0	1.2	27*
¼ cup soy protein isolate	4.2	3.2	1.0	–
½ cup wheat bran	22.0	15.4	6.6	–
1 packet sugar substitute (not aspartame)	1.0	0.0	1.0	–
RECIPE TOTAL	30.8	18.6	12.2	29
SERVING TOTAL (rounded)	5	3	2	29

* Analysis is for standard commercial mayonnaise made with soybean oil, which is rich in polyunsaturates. To increase the percentage of monounsaturated fat, use homemade mayonnaise (72 percent mono fat) or commercial canola mayonnaise.

1. Preheat oven to 375°F. Coat an 8-inch loaf pan with spray-on canola oil.
2. Combine eggs, club soda, salt, and mayonnaise in a blender. You can beat by hand with a whisk, but the blender gives a finer grain to the bread. Blend 30 seconds. Add in soy protein, wheat bran, and sugar substitute. Pour into prepared pan.
3. Bake for approximately 35 minutes.

▶ Makes 6 servings
▶ Variation: A sweet bread can be made by increasing the sweetener and adding nutmeg, vanilla, cinnamon, cloves, etc. When the bread is baked, brush with melted butter and sprinkle sweetener and cinnamon over the top.
▶ Variation: For a banana bread, add banana flavoring and walnuts. Sprinkle sweetener and ground cinnamon over the top when baked.
▶ See page 218 for more detailed nutrient contents per serving.

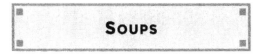

SOUPS

Broccoli Soup

YIELD IS 1 SERVING, SERVING SIZE IS 1 SERVING

INGREDIENT	CARBS, GRAMS	FIBER, GRAMS	NET CARBS	% MONO
1 cup water (or chicken stock)	0.0	0.0	0.0	–
2 tablespoons cream cheese (1 ounce)	0.8	0.0	0.8	30
¼ cup cheddar cheese (1 ounce)	0.4	0.0	0.4	33
2 tablespoons heavy cream	0.8	0.0	0.8	27
1 cup chopped broccoli	7.5	4.7	2.8	–
¼ teaspoon cumin	0.2	0.1	0.1	–
Salt and pepper (optional)	–	–	–	–
Grated Parmesan cheese (optional)	–	–	–	–
RECIPE TOTAL	9.7	4.8	4.9	29
SERVING TOTAL (rounded)	10	5	5	29

1. Steam the broccoli until tender. Add the tender broccoli to the cheeses, broth, and cumin in an electric blender, or use a hand blender. Add salt and pepper to taste. Bring to a boil to melt the cheese. Serve piping hot, adding the cream at the table. An optional sprinkle of grated Parmesan or Romano cheese completes the soup.

▶ Makes 1 large serving
▶ You can use chicken stock instead of water for a richer soup. Depending on whether you choose homemade or regular canned or fat-free broth, the amount of fats in the recipe will differ.
▶ Serve with a tossed salad with an olive oil and vinegar dressing to balance out the monounsaturated and saturated fats and also make it a satisfying lunch.
▶ See page 219 for more detailed nutrient contents per serving.

Dr. Goldberg's Chicken Soup

YIELD IS 6 SERVINGS, SERVING SIZE IS 1 BOWL

INGREDIENT	CARBS, GRAMS	FIBER, GRAMS	NET CARBS	% MONO
3 celery stalks	7.3	3.4	3.9	–
1 medium carrot	6.2	1.9	4.3	–
5 sprigs parsley	0.3	0.2	0.1	–
10 okra	9.1	3.1	6.0	–
3-pound roasting chicken	0.0	0.0	0.0	38
1 tablespoon salt	0.0	0.0	0.0	–
1 teaspoon pepper	1.4	0.6	0.8	–
RECIPE TOTAL	24.3	9.2	15.1	38
SERVING TOTAL (rounded)	4	2	2	38

1. Coarsely chop celery, carrot, parsley, and okra.
2. Wash and cut up chicken. Remove and discard the skin from the backs, thighs, and breast as well as any pieces of fat on the chicken. Place everything in a 6-quart pressure cooker. Add salt and pepper and enough water to fill the pot no more than two-thirds full.
3. Close lid and place on high heat until full pressure is reached, following instructions of your cooker. Lower the heat and cook at full pressure for 20 minutes. Remove the pot from the heat and allow to cool until the pressure has fallen. Then open the pot and remove the chicken.
4. Serve the broth with the vegetables and finely shredded, slightly cooked green cabbage as a noodle substitute.

▶ Makes about 6 to 8 bowls, depending on the amount of water you add
▶ Complete meal with chicken and a mixed vegetable salad served on the side
▶ The meat from the chicken can be eaten as a main course or, when cold, can be made into a salad or patties.
▶ If the chicken meat is later used for chicken salad, you can create two meals at once.
▶ You can make the soup without a pressure cooker, but the pressure cooker reduces the cooking time.
▶ Leftovers freeze well.
▶ See page 219 for more detailed nutrient contents per serving.

Impossibly Quick Cream of Cauliflower Soup

YIELD IS 2 SERVINGS, SERVING SIZE IS 1 SERVING

INGREDIENT	CARBS, GRAMS	FIBER, GRAMS	NET CARBS	% MONO
1 14-ounce can chicken broth	1.7	0.0	1.7	–
4 ounces half-and-half (or milk)	5.2	0.0	5.2	29
4 ounces shredded cheddar cheese (1 cup)	1.6	0.0	1.6	29
Noncarb soup thickener as desired	–	–	–	–
1 10-ounce package frozen cauliflower, cooked and drained	9.9	7.0	2.9	–
Salt and pepper to taste	–	–	–	–
RECIPE TOTAL	18.4	7.0	11.4	28
SERVING TOTAL (rounded)	9	3	6	28

1. Combine chicken broth and half-and-half and heat to simmer. Add cheese until it melts.
2. Thicken soup to desired texture with noncarb soup thickener (psyllium powder, guar gum). Add cooked cauliflower florets and heat through.

▶ Makes 2 to 3 servings
▶ Variation: Substitute cooked chopped broccoli for cauliflower and have Cream of Broccoli Soup.
▶ Variation: Use vegetable broth and soy cheese and milk and the recipe is vegan friendly.
▶ The soup thickeners will add beneficial soluble fiber.
▶ Substantive dinner-in-a-bowl with a crisp vegetable salad and an olive oil dressing.
▶ See page 219 for more detailed nutrient contents per serving.

Impossibly Quick Sauerkraut Soup

YIELD IS 4 SERVINGS, SERVING SIZE IS 1 SERVING

INGREDIENT	CARBS, GRAMS	FIBER, GRAMS	NET CARBS	% MONO
1 package dried onion soup mix	17.1	3.3	13.8	58
1 14½-ounce can of sauerkraut	17.6	10.4	7.2	—
1 14½-ounce can of crushed tomatoes, drained	33.6	9.4	24.2	—
1 teaspoon garlic powder	2.0	0.3	1.7	—
¼ teaspoon pepper	0.3	0.1	0.2	—
RECIPE TOTAL	70.6	23.5	47.1	58
SERVING TOTAL (rounded)	18	6	12	58

1. Prepare onion soup according to package. Add drained sauerkraut and tomatoes. Bring to boil, then reduce heat and simmer about 20 minutes. Add garlic powder and pepper.

▶ Makes 4 to 6 servings
▶ Good main course with a salad and cheese cubes
▶ Vegetarian friendly
▶ Great for cold winter nights
▶ You can omit or vary the amount of spices to taste.
▶ See page 219 for more detailed nutrient contents per serving.

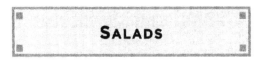

SALADS

Greek Salad

YIELD IS 4 SERVINGS, SERVING SIZE IS 1 SERVING

INGREDIENT	CARBS, GRAMS	FIBER, GRAMS	NET CARBS	% MONO
1 medium head iceberg lettuce (or mixed greens)	11.3	7.5	3.8	–
2 large tomatoes, cut in wedges*	17.0	4.0	13.0	–
1 cup Greek (Kalamata) olives	3.9	2.0	1.9	74
1 cucumber, sliced	8.1	2.2	5.9	–
1 medium onion, sliced	13.8	2.9	10.9	–
2 tablespoons olive oil	0.0	0.0	0.0	74
½ teaspoon oregano	0.5	0.3	0.2	–
2 tablespoons lemon juice (or vinegar)	2.0	0.2	1.8	–
Salt and pepper to taste	–	–	–	–
1 2-ounce can anchovies	0.0	0.0	0.0	39
4 ounces feta cheese	4.8	0.0	4.8	22
RECIPE TOTAL	61.4	19.1	42.3	49
SERVING TOTAL (rounded)	15	5	10	49

* Make sure you don't eat more than ½ cup of tomato.

1. Prepare lettuce and vegetables in bowl. Dress with olive oil. Sprinkle with oregano, lemon juice or vinegar, and salt and pepper to taste. Top with anchovy slices and feta cheese.

▶ Makes 4 servings
▶ Vegetarian friendly
▶ Main course lunch or side salad
▶ To save time, use bagged, cut-up lettuce. Slice onions and cucumbers in advance and store them in resealable bags. Olives can be stored in plastic containers in the refrigerator.
▶ See page 220 for more detailed nutrient contents per serving.

French Salade Niçoise

INGREDIENT	CARBS, GRAMS	FIBER, GRAMS	NET CARBS	% MONO
6 ounces fresh green beans cooked and then chilled	11.3	4.6	6.7	—
1 small head Boston lettuce	3.8	1.6	2.2	—
½ medium tomato	2.9	0.7	2.2	—
4 Niçoise or black olives or 1 teaspoon chopped; more if desired	1.1	0.5	0.6	74
1 6-ounce can tuna in oil, drained	0.0	0.0	0.0	31
2 teaspoons lemon juice	0.7	0.1	0.6	—
2 teaspoons olive oil	0.0	0.0	0.0	74
1 teaspoon capers	0.1	0.1	0.0	—
Salt and pepper to taste	—	—	—	—
RECIPE TOTAL	19.9	7.6	12.3	49
SERVING TOTAL (rounded)	10	4	6	49

1. Cook and cool green beans ahead of time.
2. On a plate, arrange a bed of shredded lettuce leaves. Place vegetables in 3 piles on top of the lettuce, leaving the center for the tuna. Whisk together the lemon juice and olive oil and dress the salad. Sprinkle capers and salt and pepper to taste.

▶ Makes 2 servings
▶ Main course or elegant luncheon entrée
▶ You can save time by using frozen whole green beans. Or cook extra beans for dinner the night before and use them on a luncheon salad.
▶ See page 220 for more detailed nutrient contents per serving.

Marinated Vegetable Salad

YIELD IS 4 SERVINGS, SERVING SIZE IS 1 SERVING

INGREDIENT	CARBS, GRAMS	FIBER, GRAMS	NET CARBS	% MONO
2 cucumbers, chopped	16.2	4.5	11.7	–
2 large green peppers, seeded and chopped	21.1	5.9	15.2	–
1 large onion, chopped	12.9	2.7	10.2	–
¼ cup olive oil	0.0	0.0	0.0	74
2 tablespoons vinegar	1.2	0.0	1.2	–
Salt and pepper to taste	–	–	–	–
RECIPE TOTAL	51.4	13.1	38.3	72
SERVING TOTAL (rounded)	13	3	10	72

1. Combine the chopped vegetables in a bowl and toss with dressing. Adjust dressing amounts according to the size of your vegetables. Add salt and pepper to taste.
2. Refrigerate until thoroughly chilled. Serve alongside any of your favorite meats.

▶ Makes 4 to 6 servings
▶ Use the larger servings when you're not having other carby veggies with the meals.
▶ This salad stores well in the refrigerator for 2–3 days.
▶ The salad is a summertime favorite when cucumbers and peppers are plentiful, even better when you grow your own and serve them fresh from the garden.
▶ See page 220 for more detailed nutrient contents per serving.

Middle Eastern Cucumbers

INGREDIENT	CARBS, GRAMS	FIBER, GRAMS	NET CARBS	% MONO
2 cucumbers	16.2	4.5	11.7	–
4 ounces plain yogurt (½ cup)	2.0	0.0	2.0	25
2 teaspoons dill weed	1.1	0.3	1.0	–
Salt and pepper to taste	–	–	–	–
RECIPE TOTAL	19.3	4.8	14.5	22
SERVING TOTAL (rounded)	5	1	4	22

1. Peel cucumbers and cut lengthwise. Scoop out seeds, then cut into slices lengthwise, then crosswise, so that you end up with about ½-inch cucumber cubes.
2. Put cucumber cubes into a bowl and add yogurt and dried dill. Add salt, pepper, and more dill according to taste.

▶ Makes 4 to 6 servings
▶ Vegetarian friendly
▶ Variation: Add garlic and mint and omit dill.
▶ This is an excellent accompaniment to grilled fish.
▶ See page 220 for more detailed nutrient contents per serving.

ENTRÉES

Greek-Style Gyros Plate

YIELD IS 2 SERVINGS, SERVING SIZE IS 1 SERVING

INGREDIENT	CARBS, GRAMS	FIBER, GRAMS	NET CARBS	% MONO
4 ounces ground beef	0.0	0.0	0.0	44
4 ounces ground lamb	0.0	0.0	0.0	41
1 teaspoon oregano	1.0	0.6	0.4	–
½ teaspoon rosemary	0.4	0.3	0.1	–
¼ teaspoon cumin	0.2	0.0	0.2	–
½ head iceberg (or other) lettuce	5.8	3.8	2.0	–
¼ onion, thinly sliced	2.2	0.5	1.7	–
1 clove garlic	1.0	0.1	0.9	–
1 container (8 ounces) plain yogurt	4.0	0.0	4.0	25
1 cucumber	8.1	2.2	5.9	–
Salt and pepper to taste	–	–	–	–
½ cup tomato wedges	4.2	1.0	3.2	–
8 Greek olives	2.2	1.1	1.1	74
RECIPE TOTAL	29.1	9.6	19.5	41
SERVING TOTAL (rounded)	15	5	10	41

1. Grill the beef and lamb with the spices. Prepare a plate of chopped lettuce and place the meat on top of the lettuce. Add onion.
2. Squeeze garlic through a garlic press into the yogurt. Add finely chopped cucumber and salt and pepper to taste. Mix well. Spoon sauce on top of meat.
3. Garnish with tomato wedges (no more than ½ cup per serving) and Greek olives.

► Makes 2 servings
► In season, add fresh mint leaves as garnish.
► Keep prepared gyro meat in the freezer for future quick dinners.
► You can sometimes buy prepared gyro meat packages, but some of these contain a lot of carbs as binders of the meat. So check labels before buying.
► See page 221 for more detailed nutrient contents per serving.

Eggplant Lasagna

YIELD IS 8 SERVINGS, SERVING SIZE IS 1 SERVING

INGREDIENT	CARBS, GRAMS	FIBER, GRAMS	NET CARBS	% MONO
1 large onion (1½ cups)	20.7	4.3	16.4	–
8 tablespoons olive oil	0.0	0.0	0.0	74
1 teaspoon oregano	0.5	0.3	0.2	–
1 teaspoon basil	0.4	0.3	0.1	–
Salt and pepper to taste	–	–	–	–
2 cans (about 15 ounces) stewed tomatoes*	56.9	6.9	50	–
2 teaspoons garlic powder	4.1	0.6	3.5	–
2 large eggs	1.2	0.0	1.2	40
1 teaspoon onion powder	1.9	0.1	1.8	–
1 large eggplant (about 1¼ pound) sliced ½-inch thick	28.0	10.5	17.5	–
1 cup wheat bran	44.0	30.8	13.2	–
8 ounces grated mozzarella cheese	4.8	0.0	4.8	31
1 cup grated Parmesan cheese (4 freshly grated ounces)	4.5	0.0	4.5	27
RECIPE TOTAL	167	53.8	113.3	52
SERVING TOTAL (rounded)	21	7	14	52

* This shows the carb and fiber counts if you use regular stewed tomatoes, which have more carbs than some other tomatoes. If you use canned diced tomatoes, the carb counts will be reduced to about 11 g of net carbs per serving. Check labels and buy the tomatoes or sauce with the fewest carbs.

1. Preheat oven to 350°F.
2. *To make sauce:* Finely chop the onion and sauté in about 6 table-spoons of the oil until translucent. Add the oregano, basil, salt, pepper, and tomatoes with the liquid from the can and 1 teaspoon of the garlic powder.
3. Beat 1 egg with 1 tablespoon water, salt, pepper, onion powder, and remaining 1 teaspoon garlic powder. Dip the eggplant slices in the egg mixture and then coat with wheat bran.

4. Lay the eggplant slices in a single layer on a baking sheet and brush with oil. Broil close to the heat for 5 minutes or until cooked. Turn, brush the other side with oil, and broil until the second side is done.

5. Make a layer with half the eggplant slices in a wide, shallow baking dish. Add half the tomato sauce and then layer in half the mozzarella and Parmesan. Repeat the layering with the second half of the ingredients.

6. Bake 20–25 minutes, until hot and bubbly. Allow to cool for about 10 minutes before cutting.

▶ **Makes 8 servings**

▶ **Vegetarian friendly**

▶ **This dish makes excellent leftovers for lunch.**

▶ **You can reduce the carb counts by using only 1 can of tomatoes and adding ½ can of water or other liquid to the sauce.**

▶ **See page 221 for more detailed nutrient contents per serving.**

Italian Sausages and Peppers

YIELD IS 2 SERVINGS, SERVING SIZE IS 1 SERVING

INGREDIENT	CARBS, GRAMS	FIBER, GRAMS	NET CARBS	% MONO
1 green, 1 red, and 1 yellow pepper	21.7	8.6	13.1	–
1 pound Italian sausage	3.0	0.0	3.0	46
1 medium onion, sliced	13.8	2.9	10.9	–
2 tablespoons olive oil	0.0	0.0	0.0	74
RECIPE TOTAL	38.5	11.5	27	50
SERVING TOTAL (rounded)	19	6	13	50

1. Prepare green, yellow, and red peppers into julienne strips. Cut sausages diagonally into 2-inch slices.
2. Pan-fry peppers and onion (can omit onion, if desired) in about half the olive oil until crisp-tender.
3. Remove from pan, add additional olive oil, and add cut sausage links. Fully cook, and then add peppers and onion back to skillet with meat. Heat through and serve.

► Makes 2 servings with leftovers
► Serve with steamed broccoli spears and spaghetti squash.
► This recipe is easy to double up, so you can freeze half for a future dinner.
► You can easily microwave leftovers for lunch.
► To reduce the carbs, omit the onion, or use less onion.
► See page 221 for more detailed nutrient contents per serving.

Mexican Shredded Pork or Beef

YIELD IS 4 SERVINGS, SERVING SIZE IS 1 SERVING

INGREDIENT	CARBS, GRAMS	FIBER, GRAMS	NET CARBS	% MONO
2-pound pork roast (or beef roast)	0.0	0.0	0.0	44
Optional chopped onions, peppers, and green chilies	–	–	–	–
1 16-ounce jar salsa (green or red)	21.8	4.8	17	–
1 head iceberg lettuce	11.5	7.7	3.8	–
16 black olives	4.4	2.2	2.2	74
1 medium tomato	5.7	1.4	4.3	–
½ cup onions, finely sliced	6.9	1.4	5.5	–
2 ounces cheddar cheese, shredded	0.8	0.0	0.8	29
RECIPE TOTAL	51.1	17.5	33.6	42
SERVING TOTAL (rounded)	13	5	8	42

1. Place boneless pork roast or beef pot roast in an oiled slow cooker or small roasting pan. Top with onions, peppers, and green chilies, if desired.
2. For slow cooker: Cover the meat with ½ jar of prepared salsa. Cook on low setting 8–10 hours.
3. For roasting pan: Preheat oven to 325°F. Cover meat with entire jar of salsa. Bake, covered, for 2–3 hours, until meat is fork-tender.
4. Remove meat and place on a platter. Using two forks, shred the meat apart.
5. Serve over a plate of shredded lettuce and "dress" as you would a taco, with chopped black olives, tomato, onion, and shredded cheese.

▶ Makes 4 to 8 servings
▶ Main course (4 servings) or side salad (8 servings)
▶ Shred extra lettuce and keep in a zipped bag in the refrigerator for quick meals in the near future.
▶ You can also serve on low-carb, high-fiber taco shells to make traditional tacos, using your favorite toppings.
▶ Or just use the meat in other pork or beef dishes.
▶ See page 221 for more detailed nutrient contents per serving.

Baked Mexican Casserole

YIELD IS 8 SERVINGS, SERVING SIZE IS 1 SERVING

INGREDIENT	CARBS, GRAMS	FIBER, GRAMS	NET CARBS	% MONO
6 slices low-carb high-fiber bread*	24.0	6.0	18.0	*
1 pound spicy pork (or turkey) sausage	2.3	0.0	2.3	44
8 ounces shredded colby–Monterey Jack cheese	8.0	0.0	8.0	29
1 4.5-ounce can green chili peppers	3.3	3.3	0.0	–
8 eggs	4.8	0.0	4.8	38
½ cup half-and-half (or milk)	5.2	0.0	5.2	29
RECIPE TOTAL	47.6	9.3	38.3	*
SERVING TOTAL (rounded)	6	1	5	*

* There are many different low-carb breads on the market, and they differ in their carb content. This analysis used the Food for Life brand. This product, with 4 grams of fat per slice, does not list the amount of monounsaturated fat. The label says there are zero grams of saturated fat.

1. Spray-oil the bottom and sides of a 13- x 9-inch baking pan. Place bread slices on bottom of pan to form a layer.
2. Crumble and brown the sausage, cooking thoroughly, and drain excess fat from the meat. Spoon the sausage evenly over the bread slices. Sprinkle the chilies over the sausage. Sprinkle cheese between layers, saving some to put on top of casserole.
3. Whisk together the eggs and liquid. Pour over the bread and sausage layers. Cover the pan with cling wrap and refrigerate overnight.
4. Next day, preheat oven to 350°F. Bake for 50–60 minutes, until puffed and browned. Slice into serving portions and garnish with additional toppings as desired.

▶ **Makes 8 servings**
▶ **Great brunch recipe**
▶ **Preassemble the night before for easy preparation.**
▶ **Possible garnishes include green or red salsa, sour cream, chopped olives, chopped tomatoes, and thinly sliced green onions. Use your imagination.**
▶ **See page 222 for more detailed nutrient contents per serving.**

Basic Quiche

YIELD IS 4 SERVINGS, SERVING SIZE IS 1 SLICE

INGREDIENT	CARBS, GRAMS	FIBER, GRAMS	NET CARBS	% MONO
3 large eggs	1.8	0.0	1.8	38
1 cup heavy cream	6.4	0.0	6.4	29
1 cup grated cheddar cheese	3.2	0.0	3.2	29
Pepper to taste	–	–	–	–
RECIPE TOTAL	11.4	0.0	11.4	29
SERVING TOTAL (rounded)	3	0	3	29

1. Preheat oven to 350°F.
2. Combine all ingredients with a whisk. Pour into a quiche or pie plate and bake for 45 minutes.

▶ Makes 4 servings

▶ Vegetarian friendly

▶ Variation: Add bacon, green onions, and Swiss cheese to make a traditional crustless quiche Lorraine.

▶ Variation: Use sausage, peppers, onions, mozzarella, spinach, feta cheese, and salsa. Be creative!

▶ You can serve the quiche topped with sour cream.

▶ This makes a fantastic quiche with leftover vegetables such as cauliflower or broccoli.

▶ To balance the fats, eat the quiche with a tossed salad with an olive oil dressing.

▶ Like most cheese dishes, this will increase your calcium intake.

▶ See page 222 for more detailed nutrient contents per serving.

Vegetable Quiche

YIELD IS 6 SERVINGS, SERVING SIZE IS 1 SLICE

INGREDIENT	CARBS, GRAMS	FIBER, GRAMS	NET CARBS	% MONO
2 cups cooked cauliflower	10.0	6.8	3.2	—
1 cup (4 ounces) grated cheddar cheese	1.6	0.0	1.6	29
4 large eggs	2.4	0.0	2.4	38
1 cup heavy cream (or half-and-half)	6.4	0.0	6.4	29
1 teaspoon salt	0.0	0.0	0.0	—
Pepper to taste	—	—	—	—
1 tablespoon olive oil	0.0	0.0	0.0	74
RECIPE TOTAL	20.4	6.8	13.6	33
SERVING TOTAL (rounded)	3	1	2	33

1. Preheat oven to 350°F.
2. Blend cauliflower, ¾ cup cheese, eggs, cream, salt, and pepper.
3. Oil a casserole dish or a 9-inch square baking pan with the oil. Pour in the blended mixture. Sprinkle the top with the remaining cheese.
4. Bake for 40 minutes. Let cool for about 10 minutes to set before eating.

► Makes 6 servings
► Vegetarian friendly
► This makes a fantastic Sunday dinner served with a tossed green salad. Use an olive oil dressing to balance the monounsaturated fats.
► You can use fresh or frozen cauliflower. The frozen usually packs more tightly so you'll get a few more carbs. Nutritional analysis is for fresh.
► This recipe freezes well.
► See page 222 for more detailed nutrient contents per serving.

Salmon Patties

YIELD IS 8 SERVINGS, SERVING SIZE IS 1 PATTY

INGREDIENT	CARBS, GRAMS	FIBER, GRAMS	NET CARBS	% MONO
1 16-ounce can salmon, including bones	0.0	0.0	0.0	30
2 large eggs	1.2	0.0	1.2	38
½ cup onion, chopped	6.9	1.4	5.5	–
¼ cup red (or yellow) pepper, chopped	2.4	0.7	1.7	–
1 stalk celery, chopped	2.3	1.1	1.2	–
2 tablespoons wheat bran	5.7	4.0	1.7	–
¼ cup olive oil	0.0	0.0	0.0	74
½ teaspoon salt	0.0	0.0	0.0	–
RECIPE TOTAL	18.5	7.2	11.3	56
SERVING TOTAL (rounded)	2	1	1	56

1. Mash all the ingredients together. Form patties. Fry in oil about 2–3 minutes on each side.

▶ Makes 8 to 10 patties
▶ Serve with tartar sauce and a tossed salad.
▶ You can make homemade tartar sauce by mixing 2 parts homemade mayonnaise with 1 part dill relish. This will add some monounsaturated fat and almost no carbs.
▶ See page 222 for more detailed nutrient contents per serving.

Spinach Pie

YIELD IS 6 SERVINGS, SERVING SIZE IS 1 SLICE

INGREDIENT	CARBS, GRAMS	FIBER, GRAMS	NET CARBS	% MONO
3 tablespoons olive oil	0.0	0.0	0.0	74
1 medium onion, chopped	13.8	2.9	10.9	—
1 package (10 ounces) frozen chopped spinach, thawed and squeezed of liquid	11.4	8.5	2.9	—
½ teaspoon salt	0.0	0.0	0.0	—
½ teaspoon pepper	0.7	0.3	0.4	—
¼ teaspoon ground nutmeg	0.3	0.1	0.2	—
15 ounces ricotta cheese	12.8	0.0	12.8	28
8 ounces grated mozzarella cheese	4.8	0.0	4.8	31
1 cup Parmesan cheese, freshly grated (4 ounces)	2.9	0.0	2.9	33
3 eggs	1.8	0.0	1.8	38
RECIPE TOTAL	48.5	11.8	36.7	40
SERVING TOTAL (rounded)	8	2	6	40

1. Preheat oven to 350°F. Spray an 8- or 9-inch pie pan with oil.
2. Add oil to a large heavy skillet over medium heat. Add onion and sauté until tender, about 8 minutes. Mix in spinach, salt, pepper, and nutmeg. Sauté until all the liquid from the spinach evaporates, about 3 minutes.
3. Combine ricotta, mozzarella, and Parmesan cheeses in a large bowl. Mix in eggs. Add spinach mixture and blend well.
4. Spoon the cheese-spinach mixture into the pie pan. Bake until the filling is set in the center and brown on top, about 40 minutes. Let stand 10 minutes before serving, and then cut into 6 pieces.

▶ Makes 6 servings
▶ Vegetarian friendly
▶ Serve with a small tossed salad with an olive oil dressing to balance the fats.
▶ If your family won't eat anything that isn't wrapped in pie dough, you can make the spinach pie in a prepared (or homemade) crust. Just don't eat the crust yourself.
▶ See page 223 for more detailed nutrient contents per serving.

Yankee Pot Roast

YIELD IS 4 SERVINGS, SERVING SIZE IS 1 SERVING

INGREDIENT	CARBS, GRAMS	FIBER, GRAMS	NET CARBS	% MONO
6 stalks celery	13.9	6.5	7.4	—
1 leek (or onion)	12.6	1.6	11	—
6 ounces baby carrots	13.7	3.0	10.7	—
2-pound boneless pot roast	0.0	0.0	0.0	43
2 tablespoons olive oil (for braising)	0.0	0.0	0.0	74
1 can (10¾ ounces) Golden Mushroom soup	25	1.2	23.8	18
RECIPE TOTAL	65.2	12.3	52.9	44
SERVING TOTAL (rounded)	16	3	13	44

1. Cut celery and leek into 3-inch pieces (or cut onion in half).
2. Spray the sides of a slow cooker with olive oil. Place carrots, celery, and leeks (or onions) on the bottom.
3. Brown both sides of the pot roast in olive oil in a skillet, and then put the pot roast on top of the vegetables in the slow cooker. Spread the contents of the can of soup over the top of the meat. Cover and set the slow cooker on low. Cook 8–10 hours.

▶ Makes 4 to 6 servings

▶ This makes a good dinner served with cauliflower and Brussels sprouts.

▶ It's a good meal to consider when you've got to be away all day at work or school or just running errands. With its easy preparation, you just assemble it and forget it.

▶ Most of the sauce in this recipe won't get eaten, so the actual carb counts are lower than shown. If you have a dog or cat, it'll probably be happy to lap up the juice.

▶ If you want to reduce carb counts even more, use ½ can of the soup with ¼ can of white wine or water.

▶ See page 223 for more detailed nutrient contents per serving.

Eggplant Parmesan

YIELD IS 4 SERVINGS, SERVING SIZE IS 1 SERVING

INGREDIENT	CARBS, GRAMS	FIBER, GRAMS	NET CARBS	% MONO
1 large eggplant	33.3	13.7	19.6	–
1 10-ounce can tomato puree	22.6	4.5	18.1	–
1 clove garlic, minced (1 teaspoon)	1.0	0.1	0.9	–
½ teaspoon oregano	0.5	0.3	0.2	–
½ teaspoon basil	0.2	0.1	0.1	–
1 egg	0.6	0.0	0.6	38
½ cup wheat bran	22.0	15.4	6.6	–
4 tablespoons olive oil	0.0	0.0	0.0	74
6 ounces mozzarella cheese	3.6	0.0	3.6	31
1 tablespoon grated Parmesan cheese	0.3	0	0.3	26
1 tablespoon dried parsley	0.7	0.4	0.3	–
RECIPE TOTAL	84.7	34.6	50.1	60
SERVING TOTAL (rounded)	21	8	13	60

1. Preheat oven to 350°F.
2. Cut eggplant into circles about ½-inch thick. Soak slices of eggplant in saltwater for 30 minutes and drain.
3. While soaking eggplant, make marinara sauce: Bring tomato puree, garlic, oregano, and basil to a boil. Reduce heat and simmer 20–30 minutes.
4. Dip slices into beaten egg. "Bread" the eggplant with wheat bran. Fry in olive oil until browned on both sides.
5. Arrange on oiled baking pan. Spoon marinara sauce on top of the eggplant. Top with shredded mozzarella and Parmesan cheeses. Sprinkle with dried parsley.
6. Bake 40–50 minutes or until thoroughly cooked and cheese is browned.

Recipes

- ▶ Makes 4 servings
- ▶ Variation: Use 4 boneless, skinless chicken breasts (whole or split, depending on your appetite) instead of eggplant.
- ▶ Eggplant version is vegetarian friendly.
- ▶ Main course with salad and broccoli spears
- ▶ You can save time by using premade low-carb marinara sauce.
- ▶ See page 223 for more detailed nutrient contents per serving.

Quick Chicken Divan

YIELD IS 4 SERVINGS, SERVING SIZE IS 1 SERVING

INGREDIENT	CARBS, GRAMS	FIBER, GRAMS	NET CARBS	% MONO
1 teaspoon olive oil	0.0	0.0	0.0	74
1 pound frozen broccoli spears, thawed	24.3	13.6	10.7	—
2 cups leftover roast chicken (or turkey)	0.0	0.0	0.0	40
1 can cream of chicken (or celery or mushroom) soup diluted with	27.5	2.5	25.0	43
½ soup can of red wine (or cream)	2.8	0.0	2.8	—
6 ounces cheddar (or Swiss) cheese, shredded	2.4	0.0	2.4	29
RECIPE TOTAL	57.0	16.1	40.9	35
SERVING TOTAL (rounded)	14	4	10	35

1. Preheat oven to 350°F.
2. In a 9- x 12-inch pan, coat the bottom and sides with olive oil. Arrange thawed broccoli spears to cover the bottom of the pan. Layer leftover chicken or turkey meat over the broccoli. Pour diluted soup over the meat. Top with shredded cheese.
3. Bake until thoroughly heated and cheese is melted and browned, about 30–40 minutes.
4. Serve with steamed cauliflower and a vegetable salad with an olive oil dressing to balance the fats.

▶ **Makes 4 servings**

▶ **Quick main course**

▶ **This is a great way to use up leftover roast chicken or turkey.**

▶ **See page 223 for more detailed nutrient contents per serving.**

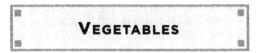

VEGETABLES

Four Corners "Mashed Potatoes"

YIELD IS 6 SERVINGS, SERVING SIZE IS 1 SERVING

INGREDIENT	CARBS, GRAMS	FIBER, GRAMS	NET CARBS	% MONO
2 large eggs	1.2	0.0	1.2	38
4 cups chopped cauliflower	20.8	10.0	10.8	–
2 tablespoons minced dried onion	8.3	0.9	7.4	–
1 cup mayonnaise*	4.9	0.0	4.9	27*
Salt and pepper	–	–	–	–
RECIPE TOTAL	35.2	10.9	24.3	27
SERVING TOTAL (rounded)	6	2	4	27

* Analysis is for standard commercial mayonnaise made soybean oil, which is rich in polyunsaturates. To increase the percentage of monounsaturated fat, use homemade mayonnaise (72 percent mono fat) or commercial canola mayonnaise.

1. Hard-boil the eggs and cool. Boil the cauliflower until overdone and soggy. Drain, mix in the onion powder, and let cool for 10 minutes.
2. Add the eggs, mayonnaise, and salt and pepper to taste, and mash all together.

▶ **Makes 6 servings**
▶ See page 224 for more detailed nutrient contents per serving.

Zucchini Latkes

YIELD IS 6 SERVINGS, SERVING SIZE IS 4 PANCAKES

INGREDIENT	CARBS, GRAMS	FIBER, GRAMS	NET CARBS	% MONO
1 large onion	12.9	2.7	10.2	—
2 pounds raw zucchini (about 8 small;	25.1	10.7	14.4	—
peel if skin is bitter)				
1 teaspoon salt	0.0	0.0	0.0	—
3 large eggs	1.8	0.0	1.8	38
¼ teaspoon pepper	0.3	0.1	0.2	—
1 teaspoon baking powder	1.1	0.0	1.1	—
1 packet sugar substitute (not aspartame)	0.9	0.0	0.9	—
⅓ cup soy flour	8.9	2.4	6.5	20
1 cup canola oil	0.0	0.0	0.0	60
RECIPE TOTAL	51.0	15.9	35.1	57
SERVING TOTAL (rounded)	9	3	6	57

1. Grate the onion and zucchini together. Add the salt and allow to drain for about 10 minutes in a colander.
2. Squeeze out the excess moisture. Add the eggs, pepper, baking powder, sweetener, and soy flour.
3. Preheat a heavy pan filled with the oil to a depth of about ¼ inch. Drop tablespoons of batter into the hot oil. Fry on medium heat for 1–2 minutes. Turn over and continue to fry until well browned.
4. Drain the pancakes on a paper towel. Serve hot with sour cream, yogurt, or kefir.

▶ Makes 6 servings, about 4 latkes per person
▶ Variation: Use olive oil instead of canola, omit the sweetener, and add a dash of tarragon.
▶ Don't reuse frying oils. If you can't bear to throw anything away, make soap.
▶ See page 224 for more detailed nutrient contents per serving.

Indian-Style Eggplant

YIELD IS 4 SERVINGS, SERVING SIZE IS 1 SERVING

INGREDIENT	CARBS, GRAMS	FIBER, GRAMS	NET CARBS	% MONO
1 large eggplant	28.4	10.7	17.7	–
4 ounces yogurt (½ cup)	2.0	0.0	2.0	25
1 teaspoon sweet curry powder (or to taste)	1.2	0.7	0.5	–
4 tablespoons chopped scallions	1.8	0.6	1.2	–
2 tablespoons olive oil	0.0	0.0	0.0	74
RECIPE TOTAL	33.4	12.0	21.4	65
SERVING TOTAL (rounded)	8	3	5	65

1. Preheat oven to 400°F.
2. Slice eggplant in half and coat cut sides with olive oil. Place oiled sides down on a baking sheet.
3. Bake 30–40 minutes until soft. Remove from oven and allow to cool before handling.
4. Scoop out eggplant and mash in a bowl. Mix with yogurt, curry spice mixture, and any remaining olive oil. Serve warm, room temperature, or chilled.
5. Top with thinly sliced green onions.

▶ Makes 4 to 6 servings

▶ For a vegetarian meal, serve with grilled vegetable kabobs for dinner.

▶ For meat lovers, serve with seasoned grilled meats or meat/vegetable kabobs.

▶ See page 224 for more detailed nutrient contents per serving.

Ratatouille

YIELD IS 6 SERVINGS, SERVING SIZE IS 1 SERVING

INGREDIENT	CARBS, GRAMS	FIBER, GRAMS	NET CARBS	% MONO
1 large eggplant	33.3	13.7	19.6	—
2 medium zucchinis	5.7	2.4	3.3	—
1 medium onion	13.8	2.9	10.9	—
1 green pepper	4.4	1.3	3.1	—
1 red pepper	7.2	2.2	5.0	—
¼ cup olive oil	0.0	0.0	0.0	74
3 cloves garlic	3.0	0.3	2.7	—
½ teaspoon thyme leaves	0.3	0.2	0.1	—
1 teaspoon basil	0.4	0.3	0.1	—
½ teaspoon oregano	0.5	0.3	0.2	—
1 can (14.5 ounces) Italian plum tomatoes, drained	8.3	1.9	6.4	—
Salt and pepper to taste	—	—	—	—
RECIPE TOTAL	76.9	25.5	51.4	71
SERVING TOTAL (rounded)	13	4	9	71

1. Cube the eggplant and zucchini. Slice onion and peppers.
2. Add olive oil to a large skillet and sauté the garlic. Over medium heat, add the cubed eggplant and zucchini. Then add the peppers and onions. Sprinkle with spices and add salt and pepper to taste.
3. Cook until the eggplant is soft and brown, adding more oil as needed.
4. Dice the tomatoes from a can of Italian plum tomatoes and add to the pot. Cook for another 10–15 minutes. Serve hot or cold as a side dish. Garnish with pine nuts and black olives if desired.

▶ Makes 6 servings

▶ This reheats well and can be frozen.

▶ You can omit the spices or use more to taste. They add almost no carbs, and many spices contain antioxidants and minerals.

▶ See page 224 for more detailed nutrient contents per serving.

Cauliflower "Rice"

YIELD IS 2 SERVINGS, SERVING SIZE IS 1 CUP

INGREDIENT	CARBS, GRAMS	FIBER, GRAMS	NET CARBS	% MONO
1 cauliflower (1 pound)	9.2	4.4	4.8	—
RECIPE TOTAL	13.8	6.6	7.2	—
SERVING TOTAL (rounded)	5	2	3	—

1. Chop cauliflower into pieces and chop in food processor until the pieces are about the size of rice. Don't process too long or it will get too watery.
2. Transfer to a glass bowl with a cover. Do *not* add water. Microwave 1 to 3 minutes until cooked, but not soft.

▶ **Makes 2 servings**

▶ **This looks like rice and makes a wonderful base for dishes with sauce.**

▶ **Add a bit of psyllium powder before cooking to add more soluble fiber and to make it a bit "stickier."**

▶ **A 1-pound cauliflower will make about 2½ cups of "rice."**

▶ **See page 225 for more detailed nutrient contents per serving.**

Sautéed Spinach

YIELD IS 4 SERVINGS, SERVING SIZE IS 1 SERVING

INGREDIENT	CARBS, GRAMS	FIBER, GRAMS	NET CARBS	% MONO
1 tablespoon olive oil	0.0	0.0	0.0	74
1 teaspoon minced garlic (or to taste)	0.5	0.0	0.5	–
½ onion, sliced thinly	4.7	1.0	3.7	–
1 10-ounce package frozen spinach	11.8	6.5	5.3	–
Salt and pepper to taste	–	–	–	–
½ teaspoon tarragon	0.2	0.0	0.2	–
RECIPE TOTAL	17.2	7.5	9.7	70
SERVING TOTAL (rounded)	4	2	2	70

1. Coat the bottom of a large sauté skillet with olive oil. Over medium heat, add minced garlic and onion to the pan, and brown.
2. Add spinach leaves and sprinkle with salt, pepper, and dried tarragon. Sauté spinach leaves until just limp, turning frequently to expose all the leaves to heat. Remove from heat and serve immediately.

▶ Makes 4 servings
▶ Variation: Use other greens.
▶ Variation: Omit tarragon and sprinkle cooked leaves with basalmic or red wine vinegar.
▶ Serve grilled salmon or scallops over sautéed spinach leaves for an elegant dinner or lunch.
▶ See page 225 for more detailed nutrient contents per serving.

Special Sprouts

YIELD IS 4 SERVINGS, SERVING SIZE IS ½ CUP

INGREDIENT	CARBS, GRAMS	FIBER, GRAMS	NET CARBS	% MONO
2 cups fresh Brussels sprouts	15.8	6.7	9.1	—
2 tablespoons olive oil	0.0	0.0	0.0	74
1 clove garlic	1.0	0.1	0.9	—
1 tablespoon lemon juice	1.0	0.1	0.9	—
RECIPE TOTAL	17.8	6.9	10.9	72
SERVING TOTAL (rounded)	4	1	3	72

1. Slice Brussels sprouts. Heat oil and fry sprouts with garlic until the sprouts are bright green. Remove from heat.
2. Add lemon juice and stir. Serve warm or cold.

▶ Makes 4 servings

▶ This makes a nice bright green addition to a meal with healthy pharmafoods and very few carbs.

▶ Brussels sprouts haters have been known to ask for seconds when they're served this way.

▶ See page 225 for more detailed nutrient contents per serving.

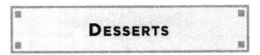

DESSERTS

Fruit Salad Dressing

YIELD IS 16 SERVINGS, SERVING SIZE IS 1 TABLESPOON

INGREDIENT	CARBS, GRAMS	FIBER, GRAMS	NET CARBS	% MONO
8 ounces plain yogurt (1 cup)	4.0	0.0	4.0	25
3 packets sugar substitute	2.7	0.0	2.7	–
6–8 drops coconut flavoring	–	–	–	–
RECIPE TOTAL	6.7	0.0	6.7	25
SERVING TOTAL (rounded)	0	0	0	25

1. Mix everything together and spoon onto cut-up fruits in individual serving cups.

▶ Makes 16 tablespoons
▶ Variation: One good mixture to serve 8–10 people is to combine 4 kiwis, 1 pint of strawberries, 1 pint of blueberries, and a quarter of a watermelon. Just make sure you don't serve yourself more than ½ cup.
▶ Variation: Use other extracts.
▶ Variation: Use other mixtures of fruits. You can even use carbier fruits if you don't serve those to yourself.
▶ Dressing can also be used as a dip with whole strawberries.
▶ Analysis is for 1 tablespoon, but this dressing has very few carbs, so you can use more than that.
▶ See page 225 for more detailed nutrient contents per serving.

Almond Macaroons

YIELD IS 24 SERVINGS, SERVING SIZE IS 1 COOKIE

INGREDIENT	CARBS, GRAMS	FIBER, GRAMS	NET CARBS	% MONO
4 egg whites	1.4	0.0	1.4	—
1 teaspoon almond extract	—	—	—	—
1 teaspoon vanilla extract	0.5	0.0	0.5	—
1 cup ground almonds	18.8	11.2	7.6	65
6 packets acesulfame-K (Sweet One or Sunette)	5.4	0.0	5.4	—
6 packets saccharin (e.g., Sugar Twin, Sweet'n Low)	5.4	0.0	5.4	—
RECIPE TOTAL	31.5	11.2	20.3	65
SERVING TOTAL (rounded)	1	0	1	65

1. Preheat oven to 350°F.
2. Beat egg whites until stiff, but not dry. Add almond and vanilla flavorings at the end of the beating. Mix the sweeteners and the nuts together, then fold in the egg whites.
3. Drop by teaspoon onto baking sheets. Bake for 20 minutes.
4. When cooled, store in an airtight plastic bag or container.

▶ Makes 24 cookies

▶ Variation: For coconut-nut macaroons, use ½ teaspoon coconut flavoring instead of almond flavoring, ½ cup chopped almonds or pecans, and 1 cup dried ground coconut. The coconut will, however, decrease the monounsaturated fat content.

▶ You may substitute 12 packets of Splenda (or ½ cup of the measure-for-measure Splenda) for the other sweeteners.

▶ See page 226 for more detailed nutrient contents per serving.

No-Bake Chocolate Cheesecake

YIELD IS 10 SERVINGS, SERVING SIZE IS 1 PIECE

INGREDIENT	CARBS, GRAMS	FIBER, GRAMS	NET CARBS	% MONO
2 ounces unsweetened baking chocolate	16.0	8.8	7.2	32
16 ounces cream cheese, softened	12.1	0.0	12.1	26
1 envelope unflavored gelatin	0.0	0.0	0.0	–
1 cup boiling water	0.0	0.0	0.0	–
1 teaspoon vanilla extract	0.5	0.0	0.5	–
18 packets sugar substitute	15.4	0.0	15.4	–
RECIPE TOTAL	44.0	8.8	35.2	29
SERVING TOTAL (rounded)	4	1	3	29

1. Melt the chocolate in a double boiler, or just microwave it with the cream cheese. Dissolve the gelatin in the boiling water in a mixing bowl. Combine all the ingredients, including the vanilla and sweetener, and stir well. Beat well with an electric mixer or place in a blender for 1 minute or until smooth.
2. Pour into muffin cups in a muffin tray. Place the muffin tray in the refrigerator and chill until firm, about 2 hours.

▶ **Makes 10 pieces**
▶ **See page 226 for more detailed nutrient contents per serving.**

Chocolates

YIELD IS 64 SERVINGS, SERVING SIZE IS 1 PIECE

INGREDIENT	CARBS, GRAMS	FIBER, GRAMS	NET CARBS	% MONO
3 ounces cocoa butter (6 tablespoons)	0.0	0.0	0.0	33
3 tablespoons butter	0.0	0.0	0.0	29
8 ounces cream cheese	6.0	0.0	6.0	28
2 tablespoons unsweetened cocoa powder	5.8	3.2	2.6	–
4 tablespoons heavy cream	1.6	0.0	1.6	27
½ teaspoon vanilla extract	0.2	0.0	0.2	–
4 tablespoons chopped walnuts	5.6	1.5	4.1	22
14 packets sugar substitute	12.6	0.0	12.6	–
RECIPE TOTAL	31.8	4.7	27.1	30
SERVING TOTAL (rounded)	0	0	0	30

1. Mix the cocoa butter, butter, and cream cheese together in a bowl over boiling water (or microwave for about 2 minutes). Stir in the cocoa.
2. Using a rubber spatula, mix in the cream, vanilla, and nuts. Stir until smooth. When the mixture is cool, add the sweetener. You may want to add more sweetener if the mixture is too bitter for you.
3. Drop onto parchment paper and refrigerate at least 2 hours, or overnight.
4. Alternatively, pour the mixture onto a nonstick cookie sheet. Cut into squares and store refrigerated.

▶ Makes 64 chocolates
▶ Variation: Use other nuts, such as macadamias, or chunky peanut butter.
▶ For "get me through the evening medicine," the dosage is 1 or 2 when you get the urge.
▶ See page 226 for more detailed nutrient contents per serving.

Peanut Butter Ice Cream

YIELD IS 6 SERVINGS, SERVING SIZE IS 1 SERVING

INGREDIENT	CARBS, GRAMS	FIBER, GRAMS	NET CARBS	% MONO
6 large eggs, separated	3.6	0.0	3.6	40
1 teaspoon vanilla extract	0.5	0.0	0.5	—
6 packets sugar substitute	5.4	0.0	5.4	—
3 tablespoons chunky peanut butter	10.4	3.2	7.2	48
½ pint heavy cream	6.4	0.0	6.4	29
RECIPE TOTAL	26.3	3.2	23.1	33
SERVING TOTAL (rounded)	4	0	4	33

1. Beat egg yolks, vanilla, and 3 packets sweetener until light in color. Stir in peanut butter until smooth.
2. Whip cream with remaining sugar substitute. Fold whipped cream into peanut butter mixture.
3. Beat egg whites until stiff peaks form and fold into mixture.
4. Pour into freezer trays or individual serving cups. Cover with transparent wrap and freeze until firm.

► **Makes 6 servings**
► **If ice cream has been in the freezer for more than 6 hours, allow to stand at room temperature for 15 minutes before serving.**
► **See page 226 for more detailed nutrient contents per serving.**

Pumpkin Pie

YIELD IS 8 SERVINGS, SERVING SIZE IS 1 PIECE

INGREDIENT	CARBS, GRAMS	FIBER, GRAMS	NET CARBS	% MONO
1 can (16 ounces) pumpkin	36.6	13.1	23.5	13
3 large eggs	1.8	0.0	1.8	38
1½ cups water	0.0	0.0	0.0	—
1 teaspoon cinnamon	1.8	1.2	0.6	—
½ teaspoon ginger	0.6	0.1	0.5	—
2 ounces crushed or ground almonds	11.6	6.2	5.4	65
1 teaspoon vanilla extract	0.5	0.0	0.5	—
½ teaspoon almond extract	0.2	0.0	0.2	—
1 tablespoon olive oil	0.0	0.0	0.0	74
8 packets saccharin (e.g., Sugar Twin)	7.2	0.0	7.2	—
8 packets acesulfame-K (Sweet One or Sunette)	7.2	0.0	7.2	—
RECIPE TOTAL	67.5	20.6	46.9	59
SERVING TOTAL (rounded)	9	3	6	59

1. Preheat oven to 450°F.
2. Oil a 9-inch pie pan and sprinkle with crushed or powdered nuts to make a crust. Blend all remaining ingredients in a blender. Pour the mixture over the nuts.
3. Bake at 425°F for 15 minutes and then at 350°F for an additional 35–40 minutes. Cool and then refrigerate.
4. Top with whipped cream sweetened with sugar substitute.

▶ Makes 8 servings
▶ You can substitute 16 packets of sucralose (Splenda) for the other sweeteners. Do not use aspartame (Nutrasweet) in this recipe.
▶ See page 227 for more detailed nutrient contents per serving.

Simple Avocado Dessert

YIELD IS 2 SERVINGS, SERVING SIZE IS 1 SERVING

INGREDIENT	CARBS, GRAMS	FIBER, GRAMS	NET CARBS	% MONO
1 ripe avocado	14.9	10.1	4.8	63
1 teaspoon lemon juice	0.3	0.0	0.3	—
1 packet sugar substitute	0.9	0.0	0.9	—
RECIPE TOTAL	16.1	10.1	6.0	63
SERVING TOTAL (rounded)	8	5	3	63

1. Cut avocado in half and remove pit.
2. Sprinkle lemon juice and sweetener on avocado and eat with a spoon.

▶ Makes 2 servings

▶ We tend to think of avocado as a vegetable, but South Americans use it in many dessert dishes. This is high in monounsaturated fat, has a creamy texture, is simple to prepare, and is delicious.

▶ See page 227 for more detailed nutrient contents per serving.

Chocolate Almond Ricotta Dessert

YIELD IS 2 SERVINGS, SERVING SIZE IS 1 SERVING

INGREDIENT	CARBS, GRAMS	FIBER, GRAMS	NET CARBS	% MONO
1 cup ricotta cheese	7.5	0.0	7.5	28
1 tablespoon unsweetened cocoa powder	2.9	1.6	1.3	—
1 packet sugar substitute (or to taste)	0.9	0.0	0.9	—
1 ounce almonds (about 22), chopped	6.9	3.9	3.0	65
RECIPE TOTAL	18.2	5.5	12.7	40
SERVING TOTAL (rounded)	9	3	6	40

1. Mix together ricotta cheese, cocoa powder, sweetener, nuts, and a few drops of almond flavoring.
2. Serve in pretty glass bowls.

▶ **Makes 2 servings**

▶ **In the summer, garnish with fresh mint leaves.**

▶ **See page 227 for more detailed nutrient contents per serving.**

Kefir Smoothie

YIELD IS 1 SERVING, SERVING SIZE IS 1 SERVING

INGREDIENT	CARBS, GRAMS	FIBER, GRAMS	NET CARBS	% MONO
½ cup plain kefir	2.0	0.0	2.0	29
½ cup unsweetened strawberries	10.1	2.3	7.8	—
½ cup ice cubes	0.0	0.0	0.0	—
1 packet sweetener	0.9	0.0	0.9	—
RECIPE TOTAL	13.0	2.3	10.7	29
SERVING TOTAL (rounded)	13	2	11	29

1. Place all ingredients in a blender and blend until smooth. You may need to add 1 tablespoon of water if it gets too thick. Pour into a tall glass and sip through a straw.

▶ Makes 1 serving
▶ Variation: Use other berries such as raspberries, blackberries, or blueberries. Carb counts vary slightly.
▶ You can buy unsweetened frozen berries that are perfect for this recipe. If you get the mixed berries, you can vary the proportions of different berries for a slightly different taste.
▶ To add more soluble fiber to your diet, add some psyllium power or guar gum to this recipe (about ½ teaspoon per cup). You may need to add a little more water if it gets too thick.
▶ See page 227 for more detailed nutrient contents per serving.

Cold Float

YIELD IS 1 SERVING, SERVING SIZE IS GLASS (6 FLUID OUNCES)

INGREDIENT	CARBS, GRAMS	FIBER, GRAMS	NET CARBS	% MONO
2 tablespoons heavy cream	0.8	0.0	0.8	29
12 ounces sugar-free soda	0.0	0.0	0.0	—
RECIPE TOTAL	0.8	0.0	0.8	29
SERVING TOTAL (rounded)	1	0	1	29

1. Add a couple of tablespoons of cream to any carbonated sugar-free drink to make a creamy float.

▶ **Makes 1 serving**

▶ **This tastes fantastic with root beer or diet chocolate fudge soda.**

▶ **See page 228 for more detailed nutrient contents per serving.**

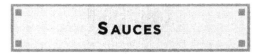

Homemade Mayonnaise

YIELD IS 24 SERVINGS, SERVING SIZE IS 1 TABLESPOON

INGREDIENT	CARBS, GRAMS	FIBER, GRAMS	NET CARBS	% MONO
2 large egg yolks	0.6	0.0	0.6	40
2 tablespoons lemon juice	2.0	0.2	1.8	–
2 tablespoons water	0.0	0.0	0.0	–
1 packet sugar substitute	0.9	0.0	0.9	–
1 teaspoon dry mustard	1.3	0.5	0.8	69
Pinch of salt	0.0	0.0	0.0	–
Dash of pepper	0.1	0.1	0.0	–
1 cup olive oil	0.0	0.0	0.0	74
RECIPE TOTAL	4.9	0.8	4.1	72
SERVING TOTAL (rounded)	0	0	0	72

1. In a small saucepan, stir all the ingredients except the oil until thoroughly blended. Cook over very low heat, stirring constantly, until mixture just starts to boil. Remove from heat and let stand for a few minutes to cool.
2. Pour into blender. Cover and blend at high speed. While blending, add oil very slowly. Blend until thick and smooth. Occasionally turn off blender and scrape down sides of container with rubber spatula.
3. Cover and chill if not used immediately.

▶ **Makes 24 tablespoons**
▶ **This recipe cooks the yolks for safety. It keeps refrigerated about 1 week.**
▶ **Use the leftover egg whites for the macaroon recipe.**
▶ **See page 228 for more detailed nutrient contents per serving.**

Alfredo Sauce

YIELD IS 37 SERVINGS, SERVING SIZE IS 1 TABLESPOON

INGREDIENT	CARBS, GRAMS	FIBER, GRAMS	NET CARBS	% MONO
2 cups heavy cream	12.8	0.0	12.8	28
3 tablespoons unsalted butter	0.0	0.0	0.0	29
1 large egg	0.6	0.0	0.6	40
¼ teaspoon pepper	0.3	0.1	0.2	–
1 tablespoon garlic (3 cloves)	2.8	0.2	2.6	–
⅓ cup Parmesan cheese, freshly grated	1.2	0.0	1.2	29
RECIPE TOTAL	17.7	0.3	17.4	29
SERVING TOTAL (rounded)	0	0	0	29

1. Pour the cream into a heavy saucepan. Add the butter and heat until warm on low heat.
2. Beat egg lightly with a fork and add to the pan. Add the pepper and garlic. Start whisking the mixture when the butter has melted. When the sauce is hot, slowly add the cheese. Raise the heat until almost boiling. Keep whisking until the sauce is smooth.
3. Remove the pot from the heat and serve the hot sauce over vegetables, eggs, or anything else you like.

▶ Makes 37 tablespoons

▶ This has a low percentage of monounsaturated fat. Eat a salad with olive oil dressing to balance the fats.

▶ See page 228 for more detailed nutrient contents per serving.

Caesar Dressing

YIELD IS 14 SERVINGS, SERVING SIZE IS 1 TABLESPOON

INGREDIENT	CARBS, GRAMS	FIBER, GRAMS	NET CARBS	% MONO
⅓ cup homemade mayonnaise	1.1	0.2	0.9	72
¼ cup Parmesan cheese	0.9	0.0	0.9	29
2 tablespoons lemon juice	2.0	0.2	1.8	—
2 tablespoons water	0.0	0.0	0.0	—
8 anchovies, chopped fine	0.0	0.0	0.0	38
½ teaspoon freshly ground pepper	0.7	0.3	0.4	—
¼ teaspoon garlic, minced (or garlic powder)	0.2	0.0	0.2	—
RECIPE TOTAL	4.9	0.7	4.2	66
SERVING TOTAL (rounded)	0	0	0	66

1. Crush the anchovies with the back of a spoon against a small bowl and then blend all ingredients together. If the dressing gets too thick, add a little water to thin it out.

▶ **Makes 14 tablespoons**
▶ **See page 228 for more detailed nutrient contents per serving.**

Yogurt Cheese

INGREDIENT	CARBS, GRAMS	FIBER, GRAMS	NET CARBS	% MONO
16 ounces plain yogurt	8.0	0.0	8.0	26
RECIPE TOTAL	8.0	0.0	8.0	26
SERVING TOTAL (rounded)	2	0	2	26

1. Put some cheescloth over a bowl. Put the yogurt into the cheese-cloth, cover the bowl, and let sit overnight in the refrigerator.
2. The next morning the cheese should be in the cheesecloth and the whey in the bowl.

▶ Makes about 8 ounces of cheese

▶ You can use a fine-mesh strainer in place of the cheesecloth. You can also buy yogurt-cheese-making kits.

▶ Farmer's cheese made from yogurt is available commercially. But it's always nicer to make your own.

▶ You can make ricotta cheese from the whey. If you're not into cheese-making, feed it to a pet.

▶ The carb counts will be even lower than shown, because much of the sugar will drain out into the whey.

▶ See page 229 for more detailed nutrient contents per serving.

Kefir or Yogurt

YIELD IS 4 SERVINGS, SERVING SIZE IS 1 CUP				
INGREDIENT	CARBS, GRAMS	FIBER, GRAMS	NET CARBS	% MONO
1 quart whole milk	45.6	0.0	45.6	28
1 ounce starter culture	0.0	0.0	0.0	—
RECIPE TOTAL	45.6*	0.0	45.6*	28
SERVING TOTAL (rounded)	11 (4)*	0.0	11 (4)*	28

* Carb counts are for the milk before culturing. After culturing, only about 4 grams of lactose (milk sugar) per cup should remain. The sourer the product, the less milk sugar is left.

1. You will have to purchase your first live-culture kefir or yogurt from a grocery store. Kefir grains can be also purchased in dried form directly from kefir manufacturers. Buy only the plain kefir or yogurt with no fruit or sugar added, and make sure it says it contains live cultures. You can eat it all except for 1 ounce (about 2 tablespoons), which you will use as a starter.

2. Place a bottle of milk in a large pot containing enough water to cover half the bottle. If you buy your milk in a carton or plastic jug, transfer it to a clean glass bottle.

3. Open the lid a little to allow for expansion of the liquid and air. Bring the water to a boil, and simmer for approximately 5 minutes. You have now pasteurized your milk. Allow the milk to cool to room temperature.

4. Add 1 ounce of kefir or yogurt to each quart of cooled milk and put the bottle top on. Mix the starter with the milk. Place the bottle on top of your refrigerator and leave it there for at least 24 hours. In cool climates you may need 36–48 hours.

5. Congratulations! You have just made a quart of kefir or yogurt. Use all of it except for the last ounce, which you will use as the starter for the next batch.

6. To eat, pour or spoon into a bowl, add sweetener, and beat with a fork for approximately 30 seconds. You will have a thick creamy liquid that you can drink or use as a topping for pancakes.

Recipes

▶ Makes 4 cups

▶ You can also make the yogurt with reduced-fat or skim milk, but it will be thinner.

▶ Two-thirds of the milk sugars will be removed by the culturing process.

▶ Homemade kefir or yogurt will keep very well for up to 2 weeks in a refrigerator. In fact, the kefir becomes smooth and creamy after about 1 week in the refrigerator, and the yogurt flavor improves.

▶ As a sauce for pancakes, mix up some kefir/yogurt with sweetener and your favorite flavoring and keep it in a glass jar to have ready when time is short.

▶ One advantage of making your own yogurt is that you have the possibility of more flavors than the same old ones you find in the grocery store. Here are some possibilities beyond the obvious vanilla, orange, lemon, cherry, banana, almond, coconut, maple, walnut, rum, and other common flavorings you can buy at the supermarket:

  ■ Pina colada: Use coconut and pineapple extracts.

  ■ Berry: Use fresh or frozen unsweetened berries thawed for approximately 40 seconds in the microwave. Zapping the fresh berries also makes the flavor more intense, as does pureeing in a small blender or food processor.

  ■ Assorted fruit flavors: Use sugar-free gelatin dessert powder as is or dissolved in a bit of water. Or use sugar-free drink mix flavorings.

  ■ Coffee: Use a teaspoon of instant coffee.

  ■ Cappuccino: Stir swirls of whipped cream into coffee yogurt and grate bitter chocolate and a little cinnamon on top.

  ■ Pumpkin pie: Use pumpkin pie spices.

  ■ Chocolate: Use cocoa powder.

  ■ Nut: Use chopped hazelnuts, almonds, or pecans with or without nut oils. Chopped nuts are also good with other flavorings.

  ■ Rosewater: Use rosewater flavoring with chopped almonds and a tiny bit of cinnamon and nutmeg. In rose season, garnish each dish with a few rose petals and a sprig of fresh mint for a dessert to serve to guests.

  ■ For special occasions, fold a little whipped cream into the yogurt.

▶ See page 229 for more detailed nutrient contents per serving.

NOTES

❖ In any of the recipes, either hot or cold, you can substitute sucralose (Splenda) for the other sweeteners. Aspartame (Equal, Nutrasweet) should not be used in recipes that are heated. The other sweeteners can be heated. When no type of sweetener is specified in an uncooked recipe, you can use any of the sugar substitutes. You will sometimes see two different sweeteners used in one recipe. This is because certain sweeteners are synergistic. This means 1 packet of each of them produces a sweeter taste and less bitterness than 2 packets of either one alone.

❖ Use your imagination to adapt the recipes to your own needs. For example, if you're on a low-salt diet, try omitting the salt and/or the baking powder in the recipes. It may not make a great deal of difference to the final product. Avoid the recipes that use salty canned soups, or substitute other ingredients.

Use full-fat or reduced-fat or low-fat dairy products, depending on your own tastes. The nutritional analyses are for full-fat dairy products (and for other ingredients like soy flour). This means the results show the "worst case" figures for saturated fat. If you use reduced-fat products, your intake of saturated fat will be lower, but so will your intake of monounsaturated fat in that product. The fat-free products usually contain more carbs and should be avoided. Read labels.

Add cheese to entrées if you need more calcium in your diet.

If you're reaching your carb limit for the meal or for the day and you're using any of the recipes in this book, scan the carb counts of individual ingredients to see if you could omit one of the carbier ingredients. For example, onions and leeks have a lot of carbs. They also taste good, but in some of the spicier recipes you could probably omit them without seeing a great change in taste. Tomatoes also have a lot of carbs. You wouldn't want to omit them in dishes like lasagna, but you could reduce the amount.

EIGHTEEN

Postscript

AT THE BEGINNING of this book, we asked you to find your personal BMI and to record it along with your weight and measurements of your waist and hips. Then we told you to put the paper with these measurements away in a drawer. If you have been on the diet for twelve weeks, it's now time to pull those measurements out and compare your present numbers with those from twelve weeks ago.

How did you do? As well as expected? Better? We told you that our study subjects lost an average of twenty pounds and five inches at the waist. But there was variability among the group.

If you lost less than this, maybe you didn't have that much to lose in the first place. We have found that once you approach your ideal body weight, this diet will keep you in balance. It will not make you lose more weight or become too skinny.

Or you may have lost fat but gained muscle. This could happen if you've been exercising. You may find your waist size went down (the waist is where we store our excess fat), but the pounds may not be as impressive. So what? You were out to lose fat. Muscle weighs more than fat.

Or maybe you are taking one of the many medications that slow down your weight loss, as described in Chapter 9. You'll still get there. It will just take longer.

Or maybe you found it hard to stay away from the carbohydrates. Why not try the diet again, but this time, do it with a friend or family member? It's always easier with support. Form your own little Four Corners Diet team and help each other with ways to break your old food habits and start good eating habits.

Be creative. Try again. You *can* do it.

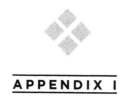

My Food Diary

YOU CAN COPY THIS FORM AND USE IT TO KEEP TRACK OF YOUR OWN FOOD
INTAKE IF YOU LIKE.

FOOD	CARBS, GRAMS	FIBER, GRAMS	NET CARBS	% MONO	COMMENTS

Recipes—
Nutrient Content per Serving

▶ Baked French Toast with Apples

NUTRIENT	QUANTITY
Calories	213
Carbohydrate	13.4 grams
Dietary fiber	2.0 grams
Net carbs	11.4 grams
Sugars	[7.0] grams
Soluble fiber	[0.3] grams
Fat	12.6 grams
Saturated fat	4.2 grams
Monounsat fat	[2.9] grams
Polyunsat fat	[0.9] grams
% mono fat	[23]
% sat fat	33
Cholesterol	224 milligrams
Protein	13.2 grams
Calcium	[63] milligrams
Magnesium	[27] milligrams
Sodium	141 milligrams
Potassium	[285] milligrams
Iron	[1.3] milligrams
Phosphorus	[149] milligrams
Vitamin A_IU	[132] IU
Vitamin C	[2.1] milligrams
Vitamin E	[0] milligrams
TAG	[19.9] grams
Glycemic Index	[18]

▶ Ricotta Pancakes

NUTRIENT	QUANTITY
Calories	251
Carbohydrate	3.5 grams
Dietary fiber	0.9 grams
Net carbs	2.6
Sugars	[0.6] grams
Fat	21.8 grams
Saturated fat	5.9 grams
Monounsat fat	11.1 grams
Polyunsat fat	3.7 grams
% mono fat	51
% sat fat	27
Cholesterol	163 milligrams
Protein	10.3 grams
Calcium	[123] milligrams
Magnesium	[31] milligrams
Sodium	89 milligrams
Potassium	[143] milligrams
Iron	[0.9] milligrams
Phosphorus	[165] milligrams
Vitamin A_IU	[201] IU
Vitamin C	[0.0] milligrams
Vitamin E	[4] milligrams
TAG	[7.3] grams

Recipes—Nutrient Content per Serving

▶ Cheese Omelet

NUTRIENT	QUANTITY
Calories	589
Carbohydrate	2.4 grams
Dietary fiber	0.0 grams
Net carbs	2.4 grams
Sugars	[2.4] grams
Fat	55.5 grams
Saturated fat	25.0 grams
Monounsat fat	22.9 grams
Polyunsat fat	3.5 grams
% mono fat	41
% sat fat	45
Cholesterol	527 milligrams
Protein	20.1 grams
Calcium	278 milligrams
Magnesium	20 milligrams
Sodium	1012 milligrams
Potassium	176 milligrams
Iron	1.7 milligrams
Phosphorus	345 milligrams
Vitamin C	0.2 milligrams
Vitamin E	[3] milligrams
TAG	[19.7] grams

▶ Fast Bran Cereal

NUTRIENT	QUANTITY
Calories	104
Carbohydrate	16.6 grams
Dietary fiber	8.3 grams
Net carbs	8.3 grams
Starch	[1.0] grams
Soluble fiber	[0.5] grams
Fat	5.2 grams
Saturated fat	0.6 grams
Monounsat fat	1.1 grams
Polyunsat fat	3.2 grams
% mono fat	22
% sat fat	12
Cholesterol	0 milligrams
Protein	5.5 grams
Calcium	30 milligrams
Magnesium	100 milligrams
Sodium	10 milligrams
Potassium	192 milligrams
Phosphorus	184 milligrams
Vitamin A_IU	0 IU
Vitamin C	0.1 milligrams
Vitamin E	1 milligram
TAG	[5.9] grams

▶ Quick Bran Pancakes

NUTRIENT	QUANTITY
Calories	309
Carbohydrate	16.3 grams
Dietary fiber	10.6 grams
Net carbs	5.7 grams
Sugars	[2.1] grams
Starch	[3.3] grams
Fat	24.4 grams
Saturated fat	4.9 grams
Monounsat fat	12 grams
Polyunsat fat	5.9 grams
% mono fat	49
% sat fat	20
Cholesterol	426 milligrams
Protein	14.6 grams
Calcium	70 milligrams
Magnesium	89 milligrams
Sodium	442 milligrams
Potassium	303 milligrams
Iron	3.5 milligrams
Phosphorus	383 milligrams
Vitamin A_IU	[10] IU
Vitamin C	15.7 milligrams
Vitamin E	[3] milligrams
TAG	27.3 grams

▶ Flax-Bran Pancakes

NUTRIENT	QUANTITY
Calories	536
Carbohydrate	26.3 grams
Dietary fiber	17.7 grams
Net carbs	8.6 grams
Sugars	[2.1] grams
Starch	[5.6] grams
Soluble fiber	[2.0] grams
Fat	40.3 grams
Saturated fat	6.4 grams
Monounsat fat	15.3 grams
Polyunsat fat	16.4 grams
% mono fat	38
% sat fat	16
Cholesterol	426 milligrams
Protein	22.9 grams
Calcium	[114] milligrams
Magnesium	[154] milligrams
Sodium	458 milligrams
Potassium	[383] milligrams
Iron	[4.2] milligrams
Phosphorus	[378] milligrams
Vitamin A_IU	[16] IU
Vitamin C	10.3] milligrams
Vitamin E	[5] milligrams
TAG	43.7 grams

Recipes—Nutrient Content per Serving

▶ Smoked Salmon Cheese Spread

NUTRIENT	QUANTITY
Calories	280
Carbohydrate	1.9 grams
Dietary fiber	0.1 grams
Net carbs	1.8 grams
Sugars	[0.3] grams
Starch	[0.0] grams
Soluble fiber	[0.0] grams
Fat	22.9 grams
Saturated fat	13.3 grams
Monounsat fat	6.7 grams
Polyunsat fat	1.6 grams
% mono fat	29
% sat fat	58
Cholesterol	84 milligrams
Protein	16.5 grams
Calcium	187 milligrams
Magnesium	21 milligrams
Sodium	210 milligrams
Potassium	245 milligrams
Iron	1.1 milligrams
Phosphorus	261 milligrams
Vitamin A_IU	[844] IU
Vitamin C	0.3 milligrams
Vitamin E	[1] milligrams
TAG	[0.5] grams

▶ Blueberry Muffins

NUTRIENT	QUANTITY
Calories	257
Carbohydrate	6.2 grams
Dietary fiber	2.0 grams
Net carbs	4.2 grams
Sugars	[2.9] grams
Starch	[0.1] grams
Fat	23.7 grams
Saturated fat	2.4 grams
Monounsat fat	14.1 grams
Polyunsat fat	6.3 grams
% mono fat	59
% sat fat	10
Cholesterol	89 milligrams
Protein	6.0 grams
Calcium	[78] milligrams
Magnesium	[46] milligrams
Sodium	105 milligrams
Potassium	[147] milligrams
Iron	[1.0] milligrams
Phosphorus	[151] milligrams
Vitamin A_IU	[8] IU
Vitamin C	[0.8] milligrams
Vitamin E	[7] milligrams
TAG	[6.3] grams
Glycemic Index value	[6]

▶ Blue Cheese Dip

NUTRIENT	QUANTITY
Calories	64
Carbohydrate	0.2 grams
Dietary fiber	0.0 grams
Net carbs	0.2 grams
Fat	6.7 grams
Saturated fat	1.5 grams
Monounsat fat	1.8 grams
Polyunsat fat	2.9 grams
% mono fat	27
% sat fat	23
Cholesterol	8 milligrams
Protein	1.1 grams
Sodium	98 milligrams
Potassium	14 milligrams
Calcium	24 milligrams
Magnesium	1 milligrams
Iron	0.0 milligrams
Phosphorus	18 milligrams
Vitamin A_IU	[30] IU
Vitamin C	0.0 milligrams
Vitamin E	[0] milligrams
TAG	1.5 grams

▶ Bread

NUTRIENT	QUANTITY
Calories	160
Carbohydrate	5.1 grams
Dietary fiber	3.1 grams
Net carbs	2 grams
Sugars	[0.6] grams
Starch	[1.1] grams
Fat	11.3 grams
Saturated fat	2.4 grams
Monounsat fat	3.4 grams
Polyunsat fat	4.6 grams
% mono fat	29
% sat fat	21
Cholesterol	148 milligrams
Protein	12.7 grams
Calcium	40 milligrams
Magnesium	33 milligrams
Sodium	288 milligrams
Potassium	111 milligrams
Iron	2.5 milligrams
Phosphorus	201 milligrams
Vitamin C	5.2 milligrams
TAG	[8.4] grams

Recipes—Nutrient Content per Serving

▶ Broccoli Soup

NUTRIENT	QUANTITY
Calories	362
Carbohydrate	9.7 grams
Dietary fiber	4.7 grams
Net carbs	5.0 grams
Sugars	[2] grams
Fat	31.4 grams
Saturated fat	18.5 grams
Monounsat fat	8.8 grams
Polyunsat fat	1.3 grams
% mono fat	29
% sat fat	58
Cholesterol	103 milligrams
Protein	14.4 grams
Calcium	345 milligrams
Magnesium	44 milligrams
Sodium	319 milligrams
Potassium	425 milligrams
Iron	2.2 milligrams
Phosphorus	274
Vitamin A_IU	[3230] IU
Vitamin C	88.2 milligrams
Vitamin E	[2] milligrams
TAG	[10.6] grams

▶ Dr. Goldberg's Chicken Soup

NUTRIENT	QUANTITY
Calories	161
Carbohydrate	4.0 grams
Dietary fiber	1.5 grams
Net carbs	1.9
Sugars	[1.4] grams
Starch	[1.0] grams
Soluble fiber	[0.6] grams
Fat	5.8 grams
Saturated fat	1.6 grams
Monounsat fat	2.2 grams
Polyunsat fat	1.3 grams
% mono fat	38
% sat fat	27
Cholesterol	64 milligrams
Protein	22.2 grams
Calcium	46 milligrams
Magnesium	36 milligrams
Sodium	1262 milligrams
Potassium	394 milligrams
Iron	1.5 milligrams
Phosphorus	191 milligrams
Vitamin A_IU	[79] IU
Vitamin C	8.7 milligrams
Vitamin E	[0] milligrams
TAG	[17.2] grams
Glycemic Index value	[13]

▶ Impossibly Quick Cream of Cauliflower Soup

NUTRIENT	QUANTITY
Calories	347
Carbohydrate	9.2 grams
Dietary fiber	3.5 grams
Net carbs	5.7 grams
Sugars	[3.7] grams
Soluble fiber	[1.0] grams
Fat	26.5 grams
Saturated fat	16.3 grams
Monounsat fat	7.4 grams
Polyunsat fat	1.0 grams
% mono fat	28
% sat fat	62
Cholesterol	84 milligrams
Protein	19.6 grams
Calcium	507 milligrams
Magnesium	38 milligrams
Sodium	1298 milligrams
Potassium	428 milligrams
Iron	1.4 milligrams
Phosphorus	406 milligrams
Vitamin A_IU	[262] IU
Vitamin C	41.7 milligrams
Vitamin E	[0] milligrams
TAG	[18.4] grams

▶ Impossibly Quick Sauerkraut Soup

NUTRIENT	QUANTITY
Calories	87
Carbohydrate	17.7 grams
Dietary fiber	5.9 grams
Net carbs	9.4 grams
Sugars	[10.2] grams
Starch	[2.2] grams
Soluble fiber	[2.2] grams
Fat	0.8 grams
Saturated fat	0.0 grams
Monounsat fat	0.3 grams
Polyunsat fat	0.2 grams
% mono fat	58
% sat fat	0
Cholesterol	1 milligrams
Protein	3.7 grams
Calcium	58 milligrams
Magnesium	43 milligrams
Sodium	1640 milligrams
Potassium	667 milligrams
Iron	2.7 milligrams
Phosphorus	91 milligrams
Vitamin A_IU	[0] IU
Vitamin C	51.4 milligrams
Vitamin E	[0] milligrams
TAG	[19.9] grams

Recipes—Nutrient Content per Serving

▶ Greek Salad

NUTRIENT	QUANTITY
Calories	239
Carbohydrate	15.3 grams
Dietary fiber	4.8 grams
Net carbs	10.5 grams
Sugars	[7.9] grams
Starch	[1.2] grams
Soluble fiber	[0.7] grams
Fat	16.2 grams
Saturated fat	5.4 grams
Monounsat fat	8.0 grams
Polyunsat fat	1.5 grams
% mono fat	49
% sat fat	33
Cholesterol	35 milligrams
Protein	10.5 grams
Calcium	232 milligrams
Magnesium	48 milligrams
Sodium	889 milligrams
Potassium	674 milligrams
Iron	2.7 milligrams
Phosphorus	202 milligrams
Vitamin A_IU	[528] IU
Vitamin C	31.2 milligrams
Vitamin E	[3] milligrams
TAG	[19.3] grams

▶ Marinated Vegetable Salad

NUTRIENT	QUANTITY
Calories	177
Carbohydrate	12.9 grams
Dietary fiber	3.3 grams
Net carbs	9.6 grams
Sugars	[5.3] grams
Starch	[0.2] grams
Soluble fiber	[0.8] grams
Fat	13.9 grams
Saturated fat	1.8 grams
Monounsat fat	9.9 grams
Polyunsat fat	1.3 grams
% mono fat	72
% sat fat	13
Cholesterol	0 milligrams
Protein	2.2 grams
Calcium	36 milligrams
Magnesium	28 milligrams
Sodium	6 milligrams
Potassium	419 milligrams
Iron	1.0 milligrams
Phosphorus	58 milligrams
Vitamin A_IU	[518] IU
Vitamin C	83.3 milligrams
Vitamin E	[4] milligrams
TAG	[9.9] grams

▶ French Salade Niçoise

NUTRIENT	QUANTITY
Calories	236
Carbohydrate	9.9 grams
Dietary fiber	3.8 grams
Net carbs	6.1 grams
Sugars	[2.2] grams
Starch	[2.8] grams
Soluble fiber	[1.0] grams
Fat	12.1 grams
Saturated fat	0.6 grams
Monounsat fat	5.9 grams
Polyunsat fat	3.4 grams
% mono fat	49
% sat fat	5
Cholesterol	24 milligrams
Protein	23.0 grams
Calcium	72 milligrams
Magnesium	60 milligrams
Sodium	430 milligrams
Potassium	750 milligrams
Iron	2.2 milligrams
Phosphorus	259 milligrams
Vitamin A_IU	[791] IU
Vitamin C	20.7 milligrams
Vitamin E	[1] milligrams
TAG	24.5 grams

▶ Middle Eastern Cucumbers

NUTRIENT	QUANTITY
Calories	41
Carbohydrate	4.8 grams
Dietary fiber	1.2 grams
Net carbs	3.6 grams
Sugars	[4.6] grams
Soluble fiber	[0.4] grams
Fat	1.2 grams
Saturated fat	0.6 grams
Monounsat fat	[0.3] grams
Polyunsat fat	[0.2] grams
% mono fat	22
% sat fat	54
Cholesterol	4 milligrams
Protein	2.2 grams
Calcium	64 milligrams
Magnesium	21 milligrams
Sodium	23 milligrams
Potassium	270 milligrams
Iron	0.7 milligrams
Phosphorus	59 milligrams
Vitamin A_IU	[64] IU
Vitamin C	8.1 milligrams
Vitamin E	[0] milligrams
TAG	[5.9] grams

Recipes—Nutrient Content per Serving

▶ Greek-Style Gyros Plate

NUTRIENT	QUANTITY
Calories	461
Carbohydrate	14.5 grams
Dietary fiber	4.9 grams
Net carbs	9.6 grams
Sugars	[12.9] grams
Starch	[0.5] grams
Soluble fiber	[1.1] grams
Fat	31.3 grams
Saturated fat	13.0 grams
Monounsat fat	12.9 grams
Polyunsat fat	2.1 grams
% mono fat	41
% sat fat	42
Cholesterol	99 milligrams
Protein	27.0 grams
Calcium	245 milligrams
Magnesium	74 milligrams
Sodium	320 milligrams
Potassium	1026 milligrams
Iron	4.6 milligrams
Phosphorus	363 milligrams
Vitamin A_IU	[272] IU
Vitamin C	24.1 milligrams
Vitamin E	[1] milligrams
TAG	[25.8] grams

▶ Eggplant Lasagna

NUTRIENT	QUANTITY
Calories	350
Carbohydrate	20.9 grams
Dietary fiber	6.7 grams
Net carbs	14.2 grams
Sugars	[8] grams
Starch	[5.8] grams
Soluble fiber	[0.9] grams
Fat	25.9 grams
Saturated fat	9.1 grams
Monounsat fat	13.5 grams
Polyunsat fat	1.9 grams
% mono fat	52
% sat fat	35
Cholesterol	89 milligrams
Protein	16 grams
Calcium	404 milligrams
Magnesium	78 milligrams
Sodium	644 milligrams
Potassium	590 milligrams
Iron	2.5 milligrams
Phosphorus	389 milligrams
Vitamin A_IU	[15] IU
Vitamin C	25.3 milligrams
Vitamin E	[3] milligrams
TAG	[32] grams

▶ Italian Sausages and Peppers

NUTRIENT	QUANTITY
Calories	983
Carbohydrate	19.2 grams
Dietary fiber	5.8 grams
Net carbs	13.4 grams
Sugars	[7.9] grams
Starch	[1.7] grams
Soluble fiber	[1.4] grams
Fat	85.1 grams
Saturated fat	26.7 grams
Monounsat fat	42.5 grams
Polyunsat fat	10.6 grams
% mono fat	50
% sat fat	31
Cholesterol	172 milligrams
Protein	35.3 grams
Calcium	75 milligrams
Magnesium	62 milligrams
Sodium	1668 milligrams
Potassium	1061 milligrams
Iron	3.8 milligrams
Phosphorus	389 milligrams
Vitamin A_IU	[3594] IU
Vitamin C	225.0 milligrams
Vitamin E	[4] milligrams
TAG	[44.6] grams

▶ Mexican Shredded Pork or Beef
(Without Optional Onion, Peppers, Green Chilies)

NUTRIENT	QUANTITY
Calories	485
Carbohydrate	12.8 grams
Dietary fiber	4.4 grams
Net carbs	8.4 grams
Sugars	6.1 grams
Starch	2.2 grams
Soluble fiber	1.2 grams
Fat	31.6 grams
Saturated fat	12.3 grams
Monounsat fat	13.4 grams
Polyunsat fat	3.1 grams
% mono fat	42
% sat fat	39
Cholesterol	126 milligrams
Protein	36.9 grams
Calcium	238 milligrams
Magnesium	59 milligrams
Sodium	629 milligrams
Potassium	968 milligrams
Iron	4.2 milligrams
Phosphorus	398 milligrams
Vitamin C	35.6 milligrams
TAG	37.4 grams

Recipes—Nutrient Content per Serving

▶ Baked Mexican Casserole

NUTRIENT	QUANTITY
Calories	358
Carbohydrate	5.9 grams
Dietary fiber	1.2 grams
Net carbs	4.7 grams
Sugars	[0.9] grams
Starch	[1.0] grams
Fat	27.0 grams
Saturated fat	11.0 grams
Monounsat fat	[8.7] grams
Polyunsat fat	[2.1] grams
% mono fat	32
% sat fat	41
Cholesterol	270 milligrams
Protein	23.4 grams
Calcium	243 milligrams
Magnesium	33 milligrams
Sodium	714 milligrams
Potassium	342 milligrams
Iron	1.6 milligrams
Phosphorus	305 milligrams
Vitamin A_IU	[357] IU
Vitamin C	10.9 milligrams
Vitamin E	[0] milligrams
TAG	[21.2] grams

▶ Basic Quiche

NUTRIENT	QUANTITY
Calories	490
Carbohydrate	2.8 grams
Dietary fiber	0.0 grams
Net carbs	2.8 grams
Sugars	2.8 grams
Starch	0.0 grams
Soluble fiber	0.0 grams
Fat	44.9 grams
Saturated fat	25.5 grams
Monounsat fat	13.2 grams
Polyunsat fat	1.9 grams
% mono fat	29
% sat fat	57
Cholesterol	302 milligrams
Protein	20 grams
Calcium	466 milligrams
Magnesium	24 milligrams
Sodium	421 milligrams
Potassium	147 milligrams
Iron	0.9 milligrams
Phosphorus	393 milligrams
Vitamin C	0.4 milligrams
TAG	18.7 grams

▶ Vegetable Quiche

(Using Fresh, Not Frozen, Cauliflower)

NUTRIENT	QUANTITY
Calories	293
Carbohydrate	3.4 grams
Dietary fiber	1.1 grams
Net carbs	2.3
Sugars	[2.6] grams
Starch	[0.3] grams
Soluble fiber	[0.3] grams
Fat	27.0 grams
Saturated fat	13.6 grams
Monounsat fat	9.0 grams
Polyunsat fat	1.4 grams
% mono fat	33
% sat fat	50
Cholesterol	217 milligrams
Protein	10.4 grams
Calcium	186 milligrams
Magnesium	15 milligrams
Sodium	568 milligrams
Potassium	148 milligrams
Iron	0.8 milligrams
Phosphorus	194 milligrams
Vitamin A_IU	[0] IU
Vitamin C	18.6 milligrams
Vitamin E	[0] milligrams
TAG	[12.3] grams

▶ Salmon Patties

NUTRIENT	QUANTITY
Calories	166
Carbohydrate	2.3 grams
Dietary fiber	0.9 grams
Net carbs	1.3 grams
Sugars	[1.0] grams
Starch	[0.4] grams
Soluble fiber	[0.2] grams
Fat	11.5 grams
Saturated fat	2.3 grams
Monounsat fat	6.5 grams
Polyunsat fat	2.0 grams
% mono fat	56
% sat fat	20
Cholesterol	84 milligrams
Protein	13.1 grams
Calcium	134 milligrams
Magnesium	28 milligrams
Sodium	211 milligrams
Potassium	259 milligrams
Iron	0.9 milligrams
Phosphorus	228 milligrams
Vitamin A_IU	[31] IU
Vitamin C	11.1 milligrams
Vitamin E	[1] milligrams
TAG	[3.6] grams

Recipes—Nutrient Content per Serving

▶ Spinach Pie

NUTRIENT	QUANTITY
Calories	409
Carbohydrate	8.1 grams
Dietary fiber	2.0 grams
Net carbs	6.1 grams
Sugars	[3.2] grams
Starch	[0.2] grams
Soluble fiber	[0.3] grams
Fat	31.0 grams
Saturated fat	15.5 grams
Monounsat fat	12.4 grams
Polyunsat fat	1.7 grams
% mono fat	40
% sat fat	50
Cholesterol	184 milligrams
Protein	25.4 grams
Calcium	640 milligrams
Magnesium	57 milligrams
Sodium	569 milligrams
Potassium	346 milligrams
Iron	2.0 milligrams
Phosphorus	460 milligrams
Vitamin A_IU	[4017] IU
Vitamin C	13.2 milligrams
Vitamin E	[2] milligrams
TAG	[15.5] grams

▶ Yankee Pot Roast
(Including Oil for Braising)

NUTRIENT	QUANTITY
Calories	739
Carbohydrate	16.3 grams
Dietary fiber	3.1 grams
Net carbs	12.3 grams
Sugars	[2.9] grams
Starch	[7.1] grams
Soluble fiber	[0.7] grams
Fat	54.3 grams
Saturated fat	19.0 grams
Monounsat fat	23.7 grams
Polyunsat fat	4.9 grams
% mono fat	44
% sat fat	36
Cholesterol	155 milligrams
Protein	44.8 grams
Calcium	77 milligrams
Magnesium	71 milligrams
Sodium	772 milligrams
Potassium	1192 milligrams
Iron	6.5 milligrams
Phosphorus	472 milligrams
Vitamin A_IU	[6325] IU
Vitamin C	13.5 milligrams
Vitamin E	[2] milligrams
TAG	[15.1] grams
Glycemic Index value	[13]

▶ Eggplant Parmesan

NUTRIENT	QUANTITY
Calories	470
Carbohydrate	21.2 grams
Dietary fiber	8.6 grams
Net carbs	12.6 grams
Sugars	[4.7] grams
Starch	[2.8] grams
Soluble fiber	[0.7] grams
Fat	38.8 grams
Saturated fat	10.5 grams
Monounsat fat	23.4 grams
Polyunsat fat	3.0 grams
% mono fat	60
% sat fat	27
Cholesterol	88 milligrams
Protein	14.4 grams
Calcium	289 milligrams
Magnesium	87 milligrams
Sodium	224 milligrams
Potassium	755 milligrams
Iron	3.1 milligrams
Phosphorus	357 milligrams
Vitamin A_IU	[1120] IU
Vitamin C	18.4 milligrams
Vitamin E	[8] milligrams
TAG	[24.1] grams

▶ Quick Chicken Divan

NUTRIENT	QUANTITY
Calories	512
Carbohydrate	14.2 grams
Dietary fiber	4.0 grams
Net carbs	10.2 grams
Sugars	[1.2] grams
Starch	[5.6] grams
Soluble fiber	[0.2] grams
Fat	24.6 grams
Saturated fat	12.4 grams
Monounsat fat	8.6 grams
Polyunsat fat	2.5 grams
% mono fat	35
% sat fat	50
Cholesterol	147 milligrams
Protein	51.5 grams
Calcium	394 milligrams
Magnesium	69 milligrams
Sodium	926 milligrams
Potassium	712 milligrams
Iron	2.8 milligrams
Phosphorus	573 milligrams
Vitamin A_IU	1620 IU
Vitamin C	77.5 milligrams
Vitamin E	[2] milligrams
TAG	[37.5] grams
Glycemic Index value	[17]

▶ Four Corners "Mashed Potatoes"

NUTRIENT	QUANTITY
Calories	318
Carbohydrate	5.9 grams
Dietary fiber	1.8 grams
Net carbs	4.1 grams
Sugars	2.4 grams
Starch	0.8 grams
Soluble fiber	[0.8] grams
Fat	32.2 grams
Saturated fat	4.8 grams
Monounsat fat	8.8 grams
Polyunsat fat	15.9 grams
% mono fat	27
% sat fat	15
Cholesterol	96 milligrams
Protein	4.4 grams
Calcium	35 milligrams
Magnesium	13 milligrams
Sodium	255 milligrams
Potassium	266 milligrams
Iron	0.7 milligrams
Phosphorus	72 milligrams
Vitamin C	32.2 milligrams
Vitamin E	[0] milligrams
TAG	11.4 grams

▶ Zucchini Latkes

NUTRIENT	QUANTITY
Calories	420
Carbohydrate	8.5 grams
Dietary fiber	2.7 grams
Net carbs	5.8 grams
Sugars	[3.9] grams
Starch	[0.2] grams
Soluble fiber	[0.9] grams
Fat	41.0 grams
Saturated fat	3.6 grams
Monounsat fat	23.6 grams
Polyunsat fat	12.1 grams
% mono fat	57
% sat fat	9
Cholesterol	107 milligrams
Protein	6.5 grams
Calcium	[105] milligrams
Magnesium	[55] milligrams
Sodium	485 milligrams
Potassium	[532] milligrams
Iron	[1.4] milligrams
Phosphorus	1172 milligrams
Vitamin A_IU	[5] IU
Vitamin C	14.6] milligrams
Vitamin E	[8] milligrams
TAG	[16.6] grams

▶ Indian-Style Eggplant

NUTRIENT	QUANTITY
Calories	112
Carbohydrate	8.3 grams
Dietary fiber	3.0 grams
Net carbs	5.3 grams
Sugars	[6.0] grams
Starch	0.1 grams
Soluble fiber	1.1 grams
Fat	8.1 grams
Saturated fat	1.5 grams
Monounsat fat	5.3 grams
Polyunsat fat	0.7 grams
% mono fat	65
% sat fat	19
Cholesterol	4 milligrams
Protein	2.2 grams
Calcium	48 milligrams
Magnesium	19 milligrams
Sodium	22 milligrams
Potassium	332 milligrams
Iron	0.7 milligrams
Phosphorus	55 milligrams
Vitamin A_IU	[63] IU
Vitamin C	2.7 milligrams
Vitamin E	[2] milligrams
TAG	[10.1] grams

▶ Ratatouille

NUTRIENT	QUANTITY
Calories	136
Carbohydrate	12.8 grams
Dietary fiber	4.3 grams
Net carbs	8.5 grams
Sugars	[4.2] grams
Starch	[1.0] grams
Soluble fiber	[0.8] grams
Fat	9.4 grams
Saturated fat	1.2 grams
Monounsat fat	6.6 grams
Polyunsat fat	0.9 grams
% mono fat	73
% sat fat	13
Cholesterol	0 milligrams
Protein	2.3 grams
Calcium	37 milligrams
Magnesium	31 milligrams
Sodium	53 milligrams
Potassium	457 milligrams
Iron	1.0 milligrams
Phosphorus	54 milligrams
Vitamin A_IU	[288] IU
Vitamin C	57.0 milligrams
Vitamin E	[2] milligrams
TAG	[15.0] grams

Recipes—Nutrient Content per Serving

▶ Cauliflower "Rice"

NUTRIENT	QUANTITY
Calories	22
Carbohydrate	4.6 grams
Dietary fiber	2.2 grams
Net carbs	1.2 grams
Sugars	2.1 grams
Starch	0.3 grams
Soluble fiber	1.1 grams
Fat	0.2 grams
Saturated fat	0.0 grams
Monounsat fat	0.0 grams
Polyunsat fat	0.1 grams
Cholesterol	0 milligrams
Protein	1.8 grams
Calcium	19 milligrams
Magnesium	13 milligrams
Sodium	27 milligrams
Potassium	268 milligrams
Iron	0.4 milligrams
Phosphorus	39 milligrams
Vitamin C	41.1 milligrams
TAG	5.7 grams

▶ Sautéed Spinach

NUTRIENT	QUANTITY
Calories	52
Carbohydrate	4.3 grams
Dietary fiber	1.9 grams
Net carbs	2.4 grams
Sugars	[1.0] grams
Starch	[1.4] grams
Soluble fiber	[0.5] grams
Fat	3.5 grams
Saturated fat	0.5 grams
Monounsat fat	2.5 grams
Polyunsat fat	0.3 grams
% mono fat	73
% sat fat	13
Cholesterol	0 milligrams
Protein	1.9 grams
Calcium	85 milligrams
Magnesium	40 milligrams
Sodium	48 milligrams
Potassium	189 milligrams
Iron	0.9 milligrams
Phosphorus	32 milligrams
Vitamin A_IU	[3] IU
Vitamin C	7.8 milligrams
Vitamin E	[1] milligrams
TAG	[5.7] grams

▶ Special Sprouts

NUTRIENT	QUANTITY
Calories	81
Carbohydrate	4.4 grams
Dietary fiber	1.7 grams
Net carbs	2.7 grams
Sugars	[0.3] grams
Starch	[0.1] grams
Fat	6.9 grams
Saturated fat	0.9 grams
Monounsat fat	5.0 grams
Polyunsat fat	0.6 grams
% mono fat	72
% sat fat	13
Cholesterol	0 milligrams
Protein	1.6 grams
Calcium	20 milligrams
Magnesium	11 milligrams
Sodium	12 milligrams
Potassium	178 milligrams
Iron	0.7 milligrams
Phosphorus	32 milligrams
Vitamin A_IU	[389] IU
Vitamin C	38.6 milligrams
Vitamin E	[2] milligrams
TAG	[1.3] grams

▶ Fruit Salad Dressing

NUTRIENT	QUANTITY
Calories	11
Carbohydrate	0.4 grams
Dietary fiber	0.0 grams
Net carbs	0.4 grams
Sugars	1.0 grams
Fat	0.5 grams
Saturated fat	0.3 grams
Monounsat fat	0.1 grams
Polyunsat fat	0.0 grams
% mono fat	25
% sat fat	63
Cholesterol	2 milligrams
Protein	0.6 grams
Calcium	[17] milligrams
Magnesium	[2] milligrams
Sodium	9 milligrams
Potassium	[22] milligrams
Iron	[0.0] milligrams
Phosphorus	[13] milligrams
Vitamin A_IU	[17] IU
Vitamin C	[0.1] milligrams
Vitamin E	[0] milligrams
TAG	0.8 grams

▶ Almond Macaroons

NUTRIENT	QUANTITY
Calories	28
Carbohydrate	1.3 grams
Dietary fiber	0.5 grams
Net carbs	0.8 grams
Sugars	0.7 grams
Fat	2 grams
Saturated fat	0.2 grams
Monounsat fat	1.3 grams
Polyunsat fat	0.5 grams
% mono fat	65
% sat fat	8
Cholesterol	0 milligrams
Protein	1.4 grams
Calcium	[10] milligrams
Magnesium	[11] milligrams
Sodium	9 milligrams
Potassium	[37] milligrams
Iron	[0.2] milligrams
Phosphorus	20 milligrams
Vitamin A_IU	[0] IU
Vitamin E	[1] milligrams
TAG	[0.9] grams

▶ No-Bake Chocolate Cheesecake

NUTRIENT	QUANTITY
Calories	198
Carbohydrate	4.4 grams
Dietary fiber	0.9 grams
Net carbs	3.5 grams
Sugars	[1.6] grams
Starch	[0.7] grams
Soluble fiber	[0.2] grams
Fat	19 grams
Saturated fat	11.8 grams
Monounsat fat	5.5 grams
Polyunsat fat	0.7 grams
% mono fat	29
% sat fat	62
Cholesterol	50 milligrams
Protein	4.6 grams
Calcium	41 milligrams
Magnesium	21 milligrams
Sodium	137 milligrams
Potassium	102 milligrams
Iron	0.9 milligrams
Phosphorus	71 milligrams
Vitamin A_IU	[647] IU
Vitamin C	0 milligrams
Vitamin E	[0] milligrams
TAG	[4.2] grams

▶ Chocolates

NUTRIENT	QUANTITY
Calories	36
Carbohydrate	0.5 grams
Dietary fiber	0.1 grams
Net carbs	0.4 grams
Sugars	[0.2] grams
Starch	[0.1] grams
Soluble fiber	[0] grams
Fat	3.7 grams
Saturated fat	2.1 grams
Monounsat fat	1.1 grams
Polyunsat fat	0.3 grams
% mono fat	30
% sat fat	56
Cholesterol	7 milligrams
Protein	0.4 grams
Calcium	[4] milligrams
Magnesium	[2] milligrams
Sodium	16 milligrams
Potassium	[10] milligrams
Iron	[0.1] milligrams
Phosphorus	[7] milligrams
Vitamin A_IU	[51] IU
Vitamin C	[0] milligrams
Vitamin E	[0] milligrams
TAG	[0.6] grams

▶ Peanut Butter Ice Cream

NUTRIENT	QUANTITY
Calories	266
Carbohydrate	4.4 grams
Dietary fiber	0.5 grams
Net carbs	3.9 grams
Sugars	[2.7] grams
Fat	23.9 grams
Saturated fat	10.8 grams
Monounsat fat	8.1 grams
Polyunsat fat	2.4 grams
% mono fat	33
% sat fat	46
Cholesterol	268 milligrams
Protein	8.9 grams
Calcium	[54] milligrams
Magnesium	[21] milligrams
Sodium	117 milligrams
Potassium	[152] milligrams
Iron	[0.9] milligrams
Phosphorus	[139] milligrams
Vitamin C	[0.2] milligrams
TAG	[8.6] grams

Recipes—Nutrient Content per Serving

▶ Pumpkin Pie

NUTRIENT	QUANTITY
Calories	116
Carbohydrate	8.5 grams
Dietary fiber	2.6 grams
Net carbs	5.9 grams
Sugars	[4.0] grams
Starch	[1.1] grams
Soluble fiber	[0.6] grams
Fat	7.4 grams
Saturated fat	1.4 grams
Monounsat fat	4.4 grams
Polyunsat fat	1.2 grams
% mono fat	59
% sat fat	19
Cholesterol	80 milligrams
Protein	4.4 grams
Calcium	[48] milligrams
Magnesium	[37] milligrams
Sodium	29 milligrams
Potassium	[196] milligrams
Iron	[1.4] milligrams
Phosphorus	[90] milligrams
Vitamin A_IU	[12490] IU
Vitamin C	[2.5] milligrams
Vitamin E	[3] milligrams
TAG	[11.5] grams
Glycemic Index value	[41]

▶ Simple Avocado Dessert

NUTRIENT	QUANTITY
Calories	164
Carbohydrate	8.0 grams
Dietary fiber	5.0 grams
Net carbs	3.0 grams
Sugars	1.3 grams
Starch	1.3 grams
Soluble fiber	[2.4] grams
Fat	15.4 grams
Saturated fat	2.4 grams
Monounsat fat	9.7 grams
Polyunsat fat	2.0 grams
% mono fat	63
% sat fat	16
Cholesterol	0 milligrams
Protein	2.0 grams
Calcium	[11] milligrams
Magnesium	[39] milligrams
Sodium	10 milligrams
Potassium	[604] milligrams
Phosphorus	[41] milligrams
Iron	[1.0] milligrams
Vitamin A_IU	[615] IU
Vitamin C	[8.5] milligrams
Vitamin E	[1] milligrams
TAG	10.7 grams

▶ Chocolate Almond Ricotta Dessert

NUTRIENT	QUANTITY
Calories	307
Carbohydrate	9.1 grams
Dietary fiber	2.8 grams
Net carbs	6.3 grams
Sugars	[0.6] grams
Starch	[1.3] grams
Fat	23.8 grams
Saturated fat	11.0 grams
Monounsat fat	9.4 grams
Polyunsat fat	2.2 grams
% mono fat	40
% sat fat	46
Cholesterol	63 milligrams
Protein	16.8 grams
Calcium	300 milligrams
Magnesium	70 milligrams
Sodium	215 milligrams
Potassium	281 milligrams
Iron	1.4 milligrams
Phosphorus	294 milligrams
Vitamin A_IU	[608] IU
Vitamin C	0.1 milligrams
Vitamin E	[1] milligrams
TAG	[7.8] grams

▶ Kefir Smoothie

NUTRIENT	QUANTITY
Calories	118
Carbohydrate	13.0 grams
Dietary fiber	2.3 grams
Net carbs	10.7
Sugars	[6.9] grams
Fat	4.1 grams
Saturated fat	2.5 grams
Monounsat fat	1.2 grams
Polyunsat fat	0.2 grams
% mono fat	29
% sat fat	61
Cholesterol	15 milligrams
Protein	4.5 grams
Calcium	[170] milligrams
Magnesium	[13] milligrams
Sodium	68 milligrams
Potassium	[164] milligrams
Iron	[0.8] milligrams
Phosphorus	[14] milligrams
Vitamin A_IU	[200] IU
Vitamin C	[46.5] milligrams
Vitamin E	[0] milligrams
TAG	20.0 grams

Recipes—Nutrient Content per Serving

► Cold Float

NUTRIENT	QUANTITY
Calories	103
Carbohydrate	0.8 grams
Dietary fiber	0.0 grams
Net carbs	0.8 grams
Sugars	0.8 grams
Starch	0.0 grams
Soluble fiber	0.0 grams
Fat	11.2 grams
Saturated fat	6.0 grams
Monounsat fat	3.2 grams
Polyunsat fat	0.4 grams
% mono fat	29
% sat fat	54
Cholesterol	41 milligrams
Protein	0.6 grams
Calcium	37 milligrams
Magnesium	6 milligrams
Sodium	86 milligrams
Potassium	30 milligrams
Iron	0.0 milligrams
Phosphorus	19 milligrams
Vitamin C	0.2 milligrams
TAG	2.2 grams

► Homemade Mayonnaise

NUTRIENT	QUANTITY
Calories	89
Carbohydrate	0.2 grams
Dietary fiber	0 grams
Net carbs	0.2 grams
Sugars	[0.1] grams
Starch	[0.1] grams
Fat	9.8 grams
Saturated fat	1.4 grams
Monounsat fat	7 grams
Polyunsat fat	0.8 grams
% mono fat	14
% sat fat	72
Cholesterol	18 milligrams
Protein	0.3 grams
Calcium	[3] milligrams
Magnesium	[1] milligrams
Sodium	4 milligrams
Potassium	[4] milligrams
Iron	0.1 milligrams
Phosphorus	[8] milligrams
Vitamin A_IU	[0] IU
Vitamin C	[0.3] milligrams
Vitamin E	[2] milligrams
TAG	[1.4] grams

► Alfredo Sauce

NUTRIENT	QUANTITY
Calories	59
Carbohydrate	0.5 grams
Dietary fiber	0.0 grams
Net carbs	0.5 grams
Sugars	[0.4] grams
Fat	6.2 grams
Saturated fat	3.4 grams
Monounsat fat	1.8 grams
Polyunsat fat	0.2 grams
% mono fat	29
% sat fat	55
Cholesterol	27 milligrams
Protein	0.8 grams
Calcium	22 milligrams
Magnesium	2 milligrams
Sodium	23 milligrams
Potassium	14 milligrams
Iron	0.0 milligrams
Phosphorus	18 milligrams
Vitamin A_IU	[6] IU
Vitamin C	0.2 milligrams
Vitamin E	[0] milligrams
TAG	[1.2] grams

► Caesar Dressing

NUTRIENT	QUANTITY
Calories	49
Carbohydrate	0.4 grams
Dietary fiber	0.0 grams
Net carbs	0.4 grams
Sugars	[0.1] grams
Starch	[0.1] grams
Fat	4.6 grams
Saturated fat	0.9 grams
Monounsat fat	3 grams
Polyunsat fat	0.4 grams
% mono fat	66
% sat fat	20
Cholesterol	10 milligrams
Protein	1.5 grams
Calcium	32 milligrams
Magnesium	3 milligrams
Sodium	119 milligrams
Potassium	19 milligrams
Iron	0.2 milligrams
Phosphorus	24 milligrams
Vitamin A_IU	[13] IU
Vitamin C	0.7 milligrams
Vitamin E	[1] milligrams
TAG	[1.1] grams

Recipes—Nutrient Content per Serving

▶ Yogurt Cheese

NUTRIENT	QUANTITY
Calories	80
Carbohydrate	2.0 grams
Dietary fiber	0.0 grams
Net carbs	2.0 grams
Sugars	6.5 grams
Fat	4.0 grams
Saturated fat	2.5 grams
Monounsat fat	1.0 grams
Polyunsat fat	0.1 grams
% mono fat	26
% sat fat	63
Cholesterol	17 milligrams
Protein	4.5 grams
Calcium	137 milligrams
Magnesium	14 milligrams
Sodium	75 milligrams
Potassium	176 milligrams
Iron	0.1 milligrams
Phosphorus	108 milligrams
Vitamin A_IU	140 IU
Vitamin C	0.6 milligrams
Vitamin E	0 milligrams
TAG	5.0 grams

▶ Kefir or Yogurt

NUTRIENT	QUANTITY
Calories	150
Carbohydrate	11.4 (4)* grams
Dietary fiber	0.0 grams
Net carbs	11.4 (4)* grams
Sugars	11.4 (4)*grams
Starch	0.0 grams
Soluble fiber	0.0 grams
Fat	8.1 grams
Saturated fat	5.0 grams
Monounsat fat	2.3 grams
Polyunsat fat	0.3 grams
% mono fat	28
% sat fat	63
Cholesterol	33 milligrams
Protein	8.0 grams
Calcium	291 milligrams
Magnesium	33 milligrams
Sodium	120 milligrams
Potassium	370 milligrams
Iron	0.1 milligrams
Phosphorus	228 milligrams
Vitamin C	2.3 milligrams
TAG	16.9 (9.5)* grams

* The computer calculates the carbs without taking into account the fact that the bacteria in the yogurt break down most of the lactose into lactic acid. Numbers in parentheses represent the corrected carb counts.

Nutritional Analysis

❖ TAG is *total available glucose*. The program totals 100 percent of the carbohydrate, 58 percent of the protein, and 10 percent of the fat in a food, because some of the protein and fat in a food can be converted to glucose by the body. This may be useful for people with diabetes who use insulin to maintain tight control of their blood glucose levels. Note that the program uses *total* carbohydrate, not the net carbohydrate content, in the calculations.

If you don't have diabetes, you don't need to worry about TAG.

❖ The brackets around the numbers in the nutritional analyses mean that at least one ingredient did not have a reported value for that nutrient in the database in the program. Hence the nutrients in brackets contain *at least* the amount specified.

❖ When the nutritional analysis simply doesn't list one of the nutrients reported for other recipes, it means that *all* the ingredients had no reported value for that nutrient. Note that having no reported value is different from having a value of zero. It simply means that the researchers didn't test for that nutrient in that food.

❖ Dashes mean that the amount of the carbohydrate, fiber, or monounsaturated fat is so small that it doesn't matter in a single serving, the ingredient is optional, or the ingredient is not included in the database. However, remember that a lot of tiny amounts can add up and affect the results for the total recipe.

❖ The percentages of monounsaturated and saturated fat in the recipe are the percentage of total fat. So if the recipe has 20 grams of fat with 10 grams of monounsaturated fat, this would be shown as 50 percent: half the fat in the recipe is monounsaturated.

This is different from the percentage of calories from fat. If a serving has 500 calories, with 20 grams of fat including 10 grams of monounsaturated fat, the monounsaturated fat would be 18 percent of the calories.

❖ Because the nutrient content per serving has been rounded off, you may get slightly different values if you use the per-serving figures to calculate monounsaturated fat percentages, especially when the amounts are small and the rounding is a significant percentage of the amount. As always, don't worry about fine points like these. The numbers are to give you a sense of the nutrient content of your food, whether a food is high or low in specific nutrients—not to tell you exactly how much there is.

❖ Be careful when you see that one serving has zero carbs, because the computer rounds anything less than 0.5 to zero. For example, the recipe for chocolates says there are zero grams of carbs per chocolate because the recipe makes so many chocolates. If you eat one or two chocolates, this isn't important. If you eat thirty-two chocolates, it is. You can always calculate the actual values by dividing the recipe total by the number of servings.

❖ Rounding off of numbers can cause differences in the reported results when the rounded numbers are used in calculations. For example, in one recipe the program reports 7 grams of mono fat in 13 grams of total fat (54 percent mono fat). If you increased the portion sizes, it would report 17 grams of mono fat in 32 grams of total fat (53 percent mono fat). If you used more decimal places, it would report 16.5 grams in 31.7 grams (52 percent). So does this recipe or ingredient contain 52, 53, or 54 percent monounsaturated fat? The answer for our purposes is, Who cares? All we want to know is that this recipe or ingredient is about half monounsaturated fat.

❖ Computer software can do amazing things with nutritional data. However, you should realize that no software can be more accurate than the data it is given to work with, and you should treat the results as close to, but not exactly matched to, reality.

Nutritional data is difficult to standardize. "One strawberry" could vary greatly in size as well as nutritional content depending on the variety of berry, degree of ripeness, soil conditions, geographical area, weather the year it was grown, and time it sat around before being eaten. USDA nutritional data are based on the "average" berry, which might not be similar to the berry you are eating. One cup of strawberries would vary in nutritional content depending on how closely you packed the berries, which would depend on their size and whether or not you sliced them up.

We have attempted to be as accurate as possible in the nutritional analyses. But one can't cover all the bases.

So don't obsess about decimal places and getting exactly the amount of the various nutrients that you want. In the long run, these small errors should balance out. Instead of weighing every morsel you eat and calculating nutritional content to four decimal places, just use estimates and *enjoy your food.*

Glossary

CALORIE A unit of energy. It is the amount of energy required to raise 1 gram of water by 1 degree Fahrenheit. Some nutritionists use the term with a capital C to mean 1,000 calories or a kilocalorie.

CARBOHYDRATES Nutritional term meaning compounds containing only carbon, hydrogen, and oxygen. They are commonly simple sugars and bigger molecules made up by joining from two to many of the simple sugars together. Examples are glucose, lactose, sucrose, maltose, starch, and glycogen. Not all carbohydrates are digestible by humans.

CHOLESTEROL A waxy sterol that is manufactured by all animal cells.

HDL High density lipoprotein—a protein and lipid particle in the blood that removes cholesterol from cells. Higher blood levels are more desirable.

HORMONE A chemical messenger secreted by one organ that influences remote tissues.

INSULIN A hormone secreted by the pancreas.

LACTOBACILLUS A lactic acid–producing bacterium that is used in the manufacture of fermented milk products. It is also a normal constituent of the intestine and the vagina.

LDL Low density lipoprotein—a protein and lipid particle in the blood that carries most of the blood's cholesterol. When damaged, it can be deposited in the artery wall. Lower values are more desirable.

LIPIDS Oily and waxy substances such as fats and cholesterol.

TRIGLYCERIDES Fat molecules composed of three fatty acids attached to a glycerol (glycerin) molecule.

VLDL Very low density lipoprotein—a protein and lipid particle in the blood whose function is to transport nondietary triglycerides around the body. Lower blood values are more desirable.

References

Diet Composition and Risk of Coronary Artery Disease

Lamarche BL, Tchernof A, et al. Fasting insulin and apolipoprotein B levels and low density lipoprotein particle size as risk factors for ischemic heart disease. *Journal of the American Medical Association* 279 (1998): 1955–61.

Maron DJ, Fair JM, and Haskell WL. Saturated fat intake and insulin resistance in men with coronary artery disease. *Circulation* 84:5 (1991): 2020–27.

Stampfer MJ, Krauss RM, et al. A prospective study of triglyceride level, low density particle diameter and risk of myocardial infarction. *Journal of the American Medical Association* 276 (1996): 882–88.

Diet Composition and Serum Lipids

Adler A and Holub BJ. Effect of garlic and fish-oil supplementation on serum lipid and lipoprotein concentrations in hypercholesterolemic men. *American Journal of Clinical Nutrition* 65 (1997): 445–50.

Knoop RH, Walden CE, et al. Long-term cholesterol lowering effects of 4 fat restricted diets in hypercholesterolemic and combined hyperlipidemic men. *Journal of the American Medical Association* 278 (1997): 1509–15.

References

Diet Composition and Weight Loss

Golay A, Allaz A, Morel Y, et al. Similar weight loss with low- or high-carbohydrate diets. *American Journal of Clinical Nutrition* 63 (1996): 174–78.

Mensink RP and Katan MB. Effect of a diet enriched with monounsaturated or polyunsaturated fatty acids on levels of low-density or high-density lipoprotein cholesterol in healthy women and men. *New England Journal of Medicine* 321 (1989): 436–41.

Plodkowski RA. Highlights from the North American Society for the Study of Obesity Annual Meeting: A Physician's View. October 11–15, 2003, Fort Lauderdale, Florida. *Medscape Diabetes & Endocrinology* 5:2 (2003). Available at: http://www.medscape.com/viewarticle/464409. Accessed December 10, 2003.

Safety of Low-Carbohydrate Diets

Alnasir FA and Fateha BE. Low carbohydrate diet. Its effects on selected body parameters of obese patients. *Saudi Medical Journal* 24:9 (September 2003): 949–52.

Brehm BJ, Seeley RJ, Daniels SR, and D'Alessio DA. A randomized trial comparing a very low carbohydrate diet and a calorie-restricted low-fat diet on body weight and cardiovascular risk factors in healthy women. *Journal of Clinical Endocrinology and Metabolism* 88 (2003): 1617–23.

Carter DF. Low-carbohydrate diet effective for adults. *Journal of Family Practice* 52 (7) (2003): 515–6.

Franz MJ. Protein and diabetes: much advice, little research. *Current Diabetes Reports* 2:5 (October 2002): 457–64.

Goldberg JM, O'Mara K, and Krembs K. Effect of a high monounsaturated fat, very low carbohydrate diet on weight and serum lipids. *Clinical Chemistry* 44 (Suppl 6) (1998): A158.

Diet Composition and Women's Health

Cohen LA, Zhao Z, Zang EA, Wynn TT, Simi B, and Rivenson A. Wheat bran and psyllium diets: effects on N-methylnitrosourea-induced mammary tumorigenesis in F344 rats. *Journal of the National Cancer Institute* 88:13 (1996): 899-907.

Franceschi S, Favero A, Decarli A, et al. Intake of macronutrients and risk of breast cancer. *Lancet* 347:9012 (1996): 1351–56.

References

Jeppesen J, Schaaf P, et al. Effects of low fat, high carbohydrate diets on risk factors for ischemic heart disease in postmenopausal women. *American Journal of Clinical Nutrition* 65 (1997): 1027–33.

Nicklas BJ, Katzel LI, et al. Effects of an American Heart Association diet and weight loss on lipoprotein lipids in obese, postmenopausal women. *American Journal of Clinical Nutrition* 66 (1997): 853–59.

Rexrode K, Hennekens C, Willett W, et al. A prospective study of body mass index, weight change and risk of stroke in women. *Journal of the American Medical Association* 227:19 (1997): 1539–45.

Rexrode K, Carey V, Hennekens C, et al. Abdominal adiposity and coronary heart disease in women. *Journal of the American Medical Association* 280:21 (1998): 1843–48.

Stoll B. Timing of weight gain in relation to breast cancer risk. *Annals of Oncology* 6 (1995): 245–48.

Wolk A, Bergstrom R, Hunter D, et al. A prospective study of association of monounsaturated fat and other types of fat with risk of breast cancer. *Archives of Internal Medicine* 158:1 (1998): 41–45.

Effect of Foods on Immunity

Schiffrin EJ, Brassart D, Servin AL, Rochat F, and Donnet-Hughes A. Immune modulation of blood leukocytes in humans by lactic acid bacteria. *American Journal of Clinical Nutrition* 66 (suppl) (1977): 521S–520S.

Solis-Pereya B, Aattouri N, and Lemonnier D. Role of food in the stimulation of cytokine production. *American Journal of Clinical Nutrition* 66 (suppl) (1977): 521S.

Effect of Monounsaturated Fats and Fiber on Diabetes

Campbell L, Marmot P, Dyer J, et al. The high monounsaturated fat diet as a practical alternative for NIDDM. *Diabetes Care* 17:3 (1994): 177–82.

Chandalia M, Garg A, Lutjohann D, et al. Beneficial effects of high dietary fiber intake in patients with type 2 diabetes mellitus. *New England Journal of Medicine* 342 (2000): 1392–98.

Garg A. High monounsaturated fat diets for patients with diabetes mellitus: a meta-analysis. *American Journal of Clinical Nutrition* 67 (suppl) (1998): 577S–582S.

References

Low C, Grossman E, and Gumbiner B. Potentiation of effects of weight loss by monounsaturated fatty acids in obese NIDDM patients. *Diabetes* 45 (1996): 569–75.

Hyperinsulinemia/Insulin Resistance

Folsom AR, Ma J, McGovern PG, and Eckfeldt H. Relation between plasma phospholipid saturated fatty acids and hyperinsulinemia. *Metabolism* 45:2 (1996): 223–28.

Grey N and Kipnis D. Effect of diet composition on the hyperinsulinemia of obesity. *New England Journal of Medicine* 285:15 (1971): 827–31.

Modan M, Halkin H, Almog S, et al. Hyperinsulinemia—a link between hypertension, obesity, and glucose intolerance. *Journal of Clinical Investigation* 75 (1985): 809–17.

Moller D and Flier J. Insulin resistance—mechanisms, syndromes, and implications. *New England Journal of Medicine* 325:13 (1991): 938–48.

O'Mara K, Shah U, Goldberg J, and Krembs K. Prevalence of hyperinsulinemia in obese subjects presenting for a weight loss program. *Chest* 112:3 (suppl) (1997): 76S.

Solymoss B, Marcil M, Chaour M, et al. Fasting hyperinsulinism, insulin resistance syndrome, and coronary artery disease in men and women. *American Journal of Cardiology* 76 (1995): 1152–56.

Zimmet P. Hyperinsulinemia—how innocent a bystander? *Diabetes Care* 16 (suppl 3) (1993): 56–70.

Pediatrics and Adolescents

Caprio S, Bronson M, et al. Coexistence of severe insulin resistance and hyperinsulinemia in preadolescent obese children. *Diabetologia* 39 (1966): 1489–97.

Dennison BA, Rockwell HL, and Baker MS. Excess fruit juice consumption by preschool-aged children is associated with short stature and obesity. *Pediatrics* 99 (1997): 15–22.

Division of Health Examination Statistics, Centers for Disease Control. Update: Prevalence of overweight among children, adolescents, and adults—United States, 1988–1994. *Journal of the American Medical Association* 227:14 (1997): 1111.

References

Sondike SB, Copperman N, and Jacobson MS. Effects of a low-carbohydrate diet on weight loss and cardiovascular risk factors in overweight adolescents. *Journal of Pediatrics* 142 (2003): 253–58.

Steinberger J, Moorehead C, Katch V, and Rocchini A. Relationship between insulin resistance and abnormal lipid profile in obese adolescents. *Journal of Pediatrics* 126:5 (1995): 690–95.

Willi SM, Oexmann MJ, Wright NM, Collop NA, and Key, LL Jr. The effects of a high-protein, low-fat, ketogenic diet on adolescents with morbid obesity: body chemistries and sleep abnormalities. *Pediatrics* 101 (1998): 61–67.

Probiotics

Hertzler SR and Clancy SM. Kefir improves lactose digestion and tolerance in adults with lactose maldigestion. *Journal of the American Dietetic Association* 103:5 (May 2003).

Kontiokari T, Laitinen J, Jarvi L, Pokka T, Sundqvist K, and Uhari M. Dietary factors protecting women from urinary tract infection. *American Journal of Clinical Nutrition* 77:3 (March 2003): 600–4.

Liu JR, Wang SY, Lin YY, and Lin CW. Antitumor activity of milk kefir and soy milk kefir in tumor-bearing mice. *Nutrition and Cancer* 44:2 (2002): 183–87.

Acknowledgments

T HE AUTHORS ACKNOWLEDGE the patience and support of their families throughout this project. Without their continued encouragement, this project would have been much more difficult to complete. We also acknowledge the assistance of summer research student Kevin Krembs. We acknowledge the study subjects who bravely tolerated many weigh-ins and laboratory tests. The study subjects and Kevin made quite a team; we all learned many things about clinical research in this process and we extend our thanks to them.

Index

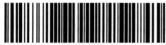

Made in the USA
Middletown, DE
28 June 2015

The Uninvited Dilemma

A Question of Gender

Revised Edition

Kim Elizabeth Stuart

Metamorphous Press
Portland, Oregon

Published by

Metamorphous Press
P.O. Box 10616
Portland, OR 97210-0616

Copyright © 1991 by Kim Elizabeth Stuart
Cover Design & Editing by Lori Stephens
Printed in the United States of America

Stuart, Kim Elizabeth
The uninvited dilemma : a question of gender /
Kim Elizabeth Stuart. - Rev. ed.
p. cm.
Includes index.
ISBN 1-55552-013-8 : $12.95
1. Transsexuals. 2. Transsexuals-Psychology. I. Title.
RC560.C4S88   1991
305.3-dc 20   91-34310